ECONOMIC EVALUATION AND HEALTH PROMOTION

For Karin, Rhian and Daniel,
and my mother, Jean

Economic Evaluation and Health Promotion

CERI PHILLIPS
Senior Lecturer in Health Economics
Department of Nursing, Midwifery and Health Care
University of Wales, Swansea

Avebury

Aldershot • Brookfield USA • Hong Kong • Singapore • Sydney

Published by
Avebury
Ashgate Publishing Ltd
Gower House
Croft Road
Aldershot
Hants GU11 3HR
England

Ashgate Publishing Company
Old Post Road
Brookfield
Vermont 05036
USA

British Library Cataloguing in Publication Data

Phillips, Ceri
    Economic evaluation and health promotion
    1. Medical economics - Great Britain
    I. Title
    338.4'7'3621

Library of Congress Catalog Card Number: 96-80385

ISBN 1 85972 487 6

Printed and bound by Athenaeum Press, Ltd.,
Gateshead, Tyne & Wear.

Contents

1. Introduction

This book has been written at a time when increasing pressure continues to mount on already stretched health care budgets; when the media abounds with accounts of rationing and its impact in health care; when health care professionals are becoming increasingly vociferous in their claims for appropriate levels of remuneration; when provider units are confronted by mounting financial pressures to meet performance targets; when purchasing agencies are faced with increasing expectations from their resident populations and there appears to be very limited scope and inclination for additional resources to be channeled into health care.

The issue of how health services should be provided and the extent of resources utilised is clearly one of the most contentious political issues of the day. However, aside from the short term political controversies there is a more fundamental issue which is taxing the minds of all governments in the developed world, namely that of longer term health policies. This is brought about as a consequence of what has been termed the health service dilemma (Phillips and Prowle, 1992), although it is part of a wider economic problem which characterises every area of the economy, and can be viewed from the individual perspective through to the global perspective. It is based on the fact that while we have unlimited wants and desires, we only have limited resources at our disposal to satisfy them. The discipline of economics emerged because of the existence of infinite demand for goods and services chasing a finite supply of resources. This situation has become particularly evident in health care and has been compounded by factors such as the increasing health needs and demands of an ageing population; continuing advancements in health technology and medical science; and, the increasing expectations of the population with regard to what can be delivered by health services.

1

At the time the NHS was formed, there was a belief that the demand for health services was finite and all that had to be done was provide sufficient financial resources and at least the majority of the health demands of the population would be satisfied. However, such a view has long since been accepted as plausible and the nature of health care is no different from any other sector of the economy. Diseases, which at one time were killers have been virtually eradicated and procedures which required long lengths of stay in hospital can now be done in GP surgeries, while new diseases and health problems have become major causes of concern for health care professionals and policy makers alike. Resources available for health services (public or private) are finite whereas the expectations of the population are continuing to increase the demands that are placed on the health care system. The question taxing the minds of governments and political parties is how to reconcile virtually infinite demand for health care and health care services with finite resources, without ending up in a position where a substantial proportion of GDP is devoted to the provision of health services, and, in all probability, still fails to meet levels of expressed demand?

A number of broad policy options have been proposed and implemented with varying degrees of success. They include schemes designed to increase efficiency by, for example, reducing the costs of catering or domestic services through competitive tendering and reducing the unit costs of treating patients by altering treatment packages from in-patient to day-case surgery; limiting the range of services provided by public providers; increasing the level of funding by levying charges, increasing taxation proceeds or shifting resources from other parts of the public sector; adopting alternative financing structures by incorporating some form of health insurance system similar to that in other European countries and the USA; adopting initiatives designed to influence the factors which affect the levels of demand for health services by, for example, health promotion schemes which emphasise responsibilities for caring for one's own health and other educational strategies; and, advocating schemes which improve the supply of health care services at similar or lower cost to the health services, through for example, implementing evidence-based practices.

One of the key policy planks of most governments has been to prevent people from becoming ill in the first place. Preventive health care and health promotion can be viewed as an attempt to focus on the factors influencing the demand for health care. Emphasising the need to take responsibility for one's own health, by not engaging in health-damaging behaviour, has been viewed as a means of alleviating the pressure on NHS resources further down the line. People adjusting their lifestyles may reduce the risk of heart disease later and the accompanying need for cardiac interventions. However, this approach displays a lack of understanding of the 'objectives of health promotion and of the role that economics can play in the pursuit of those objectives' (Cohen, 1992). Economics, as a discipline, provides a conceptual framework for assessing the extent to which health promotion activities *per se* are efficient and the relative efficiency of health promotion in terms of other health care activities. It also seeks to explain why people behave in the way they do with regard to health and what sorts of inducements need to be available to instigate a change in lifestyle.

One of the aims of this book is to demonstrate how economics can provide a framework within which priorities can be set and how economic techniques can provide an analysis of health promotion schemes in order to offer suggestions as to which schemes and programmes are relatively efficient and provide value for money for health promotion agencies and maximise the benefits to society from the resources available.

However, it should be made explicit at the outset that it is not advocated that economics and economic evaluation techniques, in and of themselves, can be used in isolation. In assessing and evaluating health promotion (and indeed any health care) policies and programmes a plurality of approaches and criteria need to be employed (Phillips et al., 1994) and it is not sufficient to utilise economic techniques as the sole basis for making decisions as to the value, or otherwise, of projects. For instance, it has been argued that 'for the purposes of an economic evaluation, equity objectives need to be clearly defined and incorporated' (Tolley, 1993). This ties in with the claim that 'in arguing their case for more resources, health promotion initiatives must have data that measure their effectiveness, efficiency, economy, quality and consumer responsiveness' (Whelan et al., 1993).

The next chapter focuses on the discipline of economics in more detail, while Chapter 3 highlights the approaches that have been used for establishing priorities and how economic techniques can be used for this purpose. Chapter 4 examines the basis for economic evaluations in health promotion and explores the methodological issues of relevance to health promotion agencies in formulating future strategies. Chapters 5 to 12 consider studies from eight areas of health promotion activity, from the perspective of methodology employed, their findings and the relevant issues for health promotion agencies. Chapter 13 draws together the main findings from each of the areas and proposes a framework for use by health promotion agencies and policy makers in developing future policies and strategies to ensure that, irrespective of the level of resources available, they are utilised in such a way as to maximise the benefits to society.

2. Introduction to economics

Economics is founded on the premise that there will never be enough resources to completely satisfy human desires. The use of resources in one activity inevitably involves a sacrifice in another (Charles and Webb, 1986). Therefore questions of resource allocation, that is how society's scarce resources are, could be or should be allocated amongst the infinite variety of competing activities, are fundamental to any study of economics and provide the rationale for an economic perspective in setting priorities. The extent of the gap which exists between the demands for commodities, such as health care and the level of resource available to meet such demands continues to frustrate politicians, professionals and policy makers alike, and the range of economic systems which have existed and evolved over time have all attempted to address the basic economic problem of allocating resources in such a way as to maximise the benefits for society. As Maynard (1994) has argued 'the issue is not whether to prioritise but how.'

Allocation of resources

An allocation of society's resources at a particular point in time, can be viewed as a complete and comprehensive description of the quantities of each and every good and service supplied or used by the government, every productive unit, every household and every distributive unit in the economy (Jones, 1979). However, such a description fails to convey the extent and complexities of the inter-relationships and processes involved in arriving at such an outcome; nor does it portray the institutional and organisational background against which such transactions take place. The diagram on p.5, figure 2.1, illustrates the complexities of a modern economy and the transactions which take place within it:

4

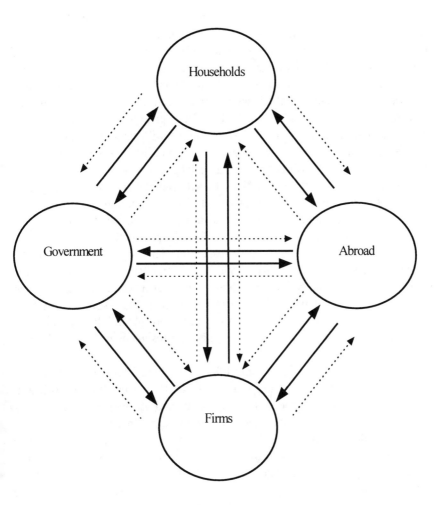

Figure 2.1: Allocation of resources in a modern economy

The diagram seeks to show that for every resource flow between agencies there is a corresponding income flow. For example, households make available human resources for firms to use in the 'production process.' In order to acquire such resources firms have to offer incentives to the households, in the form of wages and salaries. Similar transactions take place between the other agencies in the economy, all of which have a different economic impact, but add up to produce the immense number of economic engagements which occur in an economy and which result in the limited resources being allocated and distributed amongst the various agencies.

The basic aim underlying resource allocation decisions is to satisfy as many of society's needs and desires as possible within the constraints imposed by limited resources. In other words society seeks to make the most efficient use of scarce resources. The problem of *scarcity* and people's preferences force society into making *choices*, and decisions must be made as to which needs and desires are to be sacrificed in order to satisfy those needs and desires which will maximise the welfare of its members. The decision to allocate resources to a particular programme means that these resources will not be available for an alternative programmes; hence the satisfaction and utility that would be derived from these programmes will not be available. These sacrifices are referred to as *opportunity cost*. This is defined as the satisfaction that would have been gained from pursuing the next best alternative activity on a preference listing. The concept can be illustrated by reference to a situation with which one would potentially be confronted. Assume that you had decided to go to the theatre rather than to spend the evening at a restaurant. The opportunity cost of the theatre ticket is the satisfaction that would have been obtained had you spent the money on a meal at the restaurant. Thus the cost of a particular policy is the increase in welfare that would have been generated if the resources had been allocated to an alternative policy, for example, the cost of building a new ward at a hospital would be the benefits generated if the resources had been allocated to community health services.

It is thus a basic fact of economic life that nothing is free or costless and the question of whether a greater share of GNP should be devoted to health care services at the other expense of other goods and services is one which has been the subject of considerable debate and enquiry. In engaging in such a debate it should be remembered that *more* does not necessarily mean *better* health care and diverting additional resources into health care will not automatically generate an improvement in the health of the population. Economists use the term *efficiency* to consider the extent to which the allocation of limited resources maximises the benefits for society.

Efficiency

The term 'efficiency' is often misunderstood and confused with the term 'economy' and has tended to be used to describe an activity being performed at a given rate at the lowest cost. However, this is far too narrow a definition and the economic concept of efficiency embraces both inputs (costs) and outputs or outcomes (benefits). Economists have classified efficiency into various types. The simplest notion of efficiency is the one referred to above, that is to generate a given level of output at minimum cost - and is synonymous with the concept of efficiency savings, where output is expected to be maintained while at the same time making cost reductions. Efficiency, in this sense, has been referred to as technical efficiency (McGuire et al., 1988), X-efficiency (Mooney, 1986), operational efficiency (Mooney et al., 1992) and cost-effectiveness (Gerard, 1992). Technical efficiency exists when output is maximised for a given cost or where the costs of producing a given output are minimised. Allocative efficiency exists when it is impossible to make an individual better off without at the same time making someone else worse off. In order to establish priorities allocative efficiency must be utilised. In setting priorities it is not sufficient to know the most cost-effective way of treating each condition, it is necessary to decide which conditions to treat and what services to provide. Allocative efficiency, as already mentioned, is a situation where no input and no output can be transferred so as to make someone better off without at the same time making someone else worse off, a situation known as *Pareto-efficient*. However, in reality, there may well be situations where a re-allocation of resources would result in some members of society being made better off while others would be worse off. It is possible that there could be an improvement in social welfare if gainers are able to compensate losers and still be better off. This has been referred to as social efficiency and exists when 'there is no scope for potential Pareto improvement,' (McGuire et al., 1988). The criterion for social efficiency is that the amount by which the beneficiaries gain exceeds the extent to which the losers lose. This has been adapted by Drummond (1989) to 'ensuring that goods and services are allocated so as to maximise the welfare of the community,' known also as top-level or global efficiency (Coast, 1996). This presupposes that technical efficiency is present in all individual health care services.

The objective of endeavouring to maximise the benefits to society given the level of resources available appears, at first sight, to be perfectly valid and commendable. However, there are a number of other issues which impinge on the pursuit of such an objective. For example, problems arise as to *whose* valuations of appropriate compensation are to be adopted since such decisions are dependent upon the distribution of income. In reality it is impossible to separate decisions regarding resource allocation from those regarding income distribution. A move towards Pareto-efficiency may well result in a redistribution of income in favour of the well-off, which may not be acceptable on grounds of equity. For example, if the increase in income generated by a re-allocation of resources were to pass to the affluent members of society, then even though the less well-off were not made worse off, there would have been a redistribution of income in favour of the well-off as a result of the move towards efficiency. Since equity is one of the main aspects associated with social welfare then such implications cannot be ignored by policy makers in assessing the allocation of resources. The notion of equity has been discussed and debated at length in the literature (see, for example, Coast et al., 1996; Donaldson and

Gerard, 1993; Mooney, 1994; Palfrey et al., 1992; Phillips et al., 1994). Indeed, from scanning policy documents one would be excused from deducing that equity was one of the primary goals of health policy. The reality often appears to be very different with the emphasis firmly placed on efficiency, and efficiency in a very narrow sense at that.

Another important consideration is based on what constitutes the 'benefit' in assessing the efficiency of resource allocations (Mooney and Lange, 1993). The nature of health and health care makes it very difficult to assume that the benefit of health care interventions only surround the utility and satisfaction gained from receiving the services. There are other potential benefits in terms of improved health and quality of life, benefits to other family members, for example, who have been concerned because of one person's health problem.

Discussions surrounding Pareto-efficiency demonstrate that such a situation would be achieved by the 'invisible hand' of the free market, where the forces of supply and demand ensure that a single price for products enable the quantities demanded and supplied to be equal. i.e. there would be no shortages or surpluses of any commodity and no individual or firm would have any incentive to alter the pattern of consumption or production. The next section explores the concept of the market and the conditions necessary for a market to function efficiently in health care and outlines why the absence of these conditions results in what is termed *market failure*.

Market

A market for any good or service is composed of a *demand* side, based on consumers wants and desires supported by an ability to pay for the particular commodity, a *supply* side, based on producers aim to generate profit and the interaction between them. Markets operate according to price signals - if prices change then demand and supply will adjust to a position where producers are able to sell all that they want at the price and consumers are able to purchase all that they want. Similarly, if levels of demand and/or supply alter the price will adjust to reflect such changes and move to a position where demand and supply are equal. This position is referred to as *market equilibrium*, and is shown at price Pe and quantity Qe in the diagram, figure 2.2 on page 9.

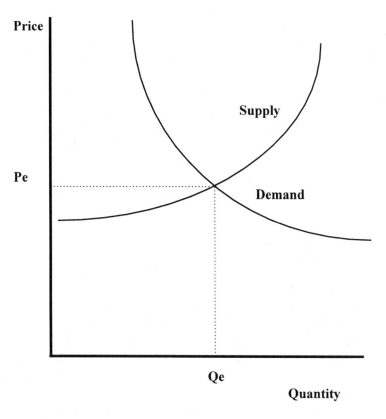

Figure 2.2: The market mechanism

In order for the market mechanism to result in a *Pareto-efficient* allocation of resources a number of conditions must apply. The first condition is the existence of perfect competition, i.e. an extremely large number of both buyers and sellers trading in a homogeneous product, with complete freedom to enter or leave the market, perfect and complete knowledge of the market and freedom of mobility for the factors of production. However, in the real world perfect competition does not exist; rather markets are characterised by monopolistic tendencies and other structures which allow individual firms to exercise considerable control over the price to be charged or the amount to be produced.

Even if perfect competition did exist there are certain types of goods which either would not be provided at all, or would be provided inadequately or in insufficient quantity by private firms. The demand side of the market mechanism is characterised by a desire for a commodity plus an ability to pay for it. For many products this may be perfectly realistic but for a range of others

9

it may not be. The characteristics of *public goods* mean that such commodities are provided by central or local government (e.g. defence, street lighting) or not at all. In addition the government intervenes to provide 'merit' goods, which would appear higher on society's preference listing than on an aggregation of individuals' preference listings, alongside private firms, e.g. education, health and transport.

Connected with market failure are the problem of *externalities*, which arise when the activities of one economic agent directly affect the outcome of the activities of another agent and are not covered by the price mechanism. Thus the noise or pollution from a factory may adversely affect the activities of a market gardener operating in close proximity to the factory, and yet no account would be taken of this by the price mechanism. It is only by the introduction of a system of compensation or legal prohibition by the government that these consequences can be adequately dealt with. Generally, private sector decisions only take into account the private costs and benefits associated with the production and consumption of commodities. The wider social costs and benefits, which accrue to anyone in society irrespective of whether or not they were involved in the transaction or activity, can only be dealt with by government intervention.

Within the real world there are very few *future markets* but resources have to be allocated now for the production of activities in the future. A firm would not build a new factory if it were not reasonably confident of being able to sell the output from that factory. However, given society's preference for current rather than future consumption, prices tend to reflect today's costs and demands. Since resources are scarce and need to be conserved for future generations, intervention may be necessary to ration supply in the short term. In addition, outcomes are far from certain and despite the existence of insurance companies the price mechanism is biased against risky activities and situations, which may be inefficient from society's perspective. For example, many developments in transport were met with considerable scepticism in their early stages and yet have shown themselves to be highly efficient, e.g. air travel.

The failure of the market mechanism to achieve an efficient allocation of resources therefore necessitates some form of government intervention in the operation of the economy. This is particularly the case in health care, where governments involve themselves to varying degrees to try and ensure that all citizens have access to health care services. Reference has already been made to the debate over the importance of equity in formulating health policy and many initiatives have tried to address the problems associated with   access, opportunities and distribution of services, etc. In constructing policy decisions there is a broad consensus that both aspects of social welfare (i.e. efficiency and equity) should be considered in the location, method and degree of government intervention in health care and there is general agreement that there is a need for a trade-off between achieving an efficient allocation of resources and ensuring that the resulting allocation is reasonably equitable. The reality of the situation is however very different, with economic pressures forcing governments to focus on efficiency as the main driving force in formulating health care policy.

Other unusual features of the health care market relate to the extent of uncertainty at all levels, the asymmetry of information and the effects of externalities. One of the necessary characteristics for perfect competition to exist is that of perfect information and knowledge of the participants and transactions occurring in the market. In health care what is evident is that levels of understanding of, for example, the causes and progression of diseases is far from certain and which treatment regimes are known to be effective in securing health care benefits (Borowitz and Sheldon, 1993). There is also a very large gulf between the knowledge of patients, providers and purchasers of health care services - the asymmetry of information. The problems associated with externalities have already been highlighted above. These are most noticeable in health care. For example, a purchasing agency would find it extremely difficult to restrict access to a health promotion programme it had purchased to only its own residents without some spillover effects into surrounding communities. Thus, given the nature of health care, virtually all health systems exist with some degree of government intervention. The operation of the market in health care and the rationale for government intervention is well documented and interested readers are recommended to refer to such texts, for example, Donaldson and Gerard (1993); McGuire et al. (1988); Phelps (1992).

What has therefore arisen is an array of health care systems with different financing structures and proportions of public funding in existence throughout the world. What has also been noticeable is that the basic economic problem of unlimited wants, desires and needs exceeding limited resources is especially prominent in terms of health care. The health care dilemma (Phillips and Prowle, 1992) of demand for health care services outstripping available resources has been and continues to be exacerbated by the increasing health needs and demands generated by ageing populations, by continual advancements in medical science and by the increasing aspirations of populations regarding health and health care services. Governments are being bombarded with stark messages from pressure groups of the consequences of not increasing the proportion of Gross National Product (GNP) allocated to health care services. Within the UK, for example, health care purchasers are confronted by increasing demands on their limited resources and are having to confront increasingly difficult decisions as to where to channel their resources and providers, also faced by pressures on resources (for example, changes in working conditions, increases in the number of emergency admissions, bed blocking as a result of resource constraints in other sectors of health and social care) are being forced to rationalise the services they provide.

11

Given the nature of the health care dilemma there are a range of policy options available to plug the gap between demands and the supply of health care services, which have been referred to earlier. They include increasing efficiency, limiting the range of services provided, allocating additional resources to the health service, introducing alternative financing structures, reducing the level of demand for health services and dealing with issues which act as constraints on the supply of services.

All of these have been introduced in a variety of shapes and forms in a number of countries, and which, to date, have been more noteworthy for their limitations and problems of implementation rather than their success in addressing the dilemma. Indeed, it is probable that the dilemma will intensify as the demand for health care services continues to increase while the pressures on public expenditure may result in a downward trend in available resources for health care services. Within the UK, for example, the reforms in health care during the early 1990s, with the disaggregation of the purchasing and providing functions in health care, have met with some successes, for example the improvements in information flows between health authorities, trusts and GP fundholders, reductions in waiting times for some treatments and the ability to generate so-called *efficiency savings*, year-on-year. However, the media contains many more reports of issues which reflect the extent of the gap between available resources and the demands being placed on such resources. The call for additional resources, at least within the UK context, is highly unlikely to result in a significant re-allocation of funds in favour of health and so what avenues are open to policy makers and managers within the health service?

Economics, as a discipline, can provide a way forward. The concepts introduced at the beginning of this chapter were *scarcity, choice and cost.* As individuals we have to make choices every day because our resources, our time and our abilities, etc. are limited. In choosing to do one thing we are simultaneously choosing not to do some other thing. In spending our money in one area we are not able to spend it in other areas. We thus have to decide on what activities to spend our time and on what products to spend our money. In making such decisions we have, either explicitly or implicitly, something akin to a preference list or set of priorities. The same principles apply in terms of health care. In order to decide how much of the limited resources available to allocate to different aspects of health care services we need some sort of priority list. The next chapter discusses some of the approaches that have been used in planning health care services and explores how economic techniques can also contribute to the decision making process.

3. Priority setting

A working party established by the Royal College of Physicians 'to consider the practical constraints placed on health care staff in meeting public expectations and to acknowledge the problems encountered both in practice' concluded that 'choices will have to be made and priorities set that take into account both the wishes of the public and the views and experience of the health care professions' (Royal College of Physicians, 1995).

In many senses the notion of having to make choices as to who receives care is not new and there have been many examples (some anecdotal) of priorities being established, albeit implicitly, through ability to pay, the management of waiting lists, the status of the GP practice, the age of the patient, political sensitivities and so on. What has been happening of late is that the nature of the health care dilemma has forced the debate into the public arena. The health care dilemma was highlighted in the previous chapter, as were the numerous policy instruments which have been used to try and remedy the problem. The range of policy options included increasing efficiency and limiting the range of services provided. If a narrow interpretation is placed on increasing efficiency, these two options are the same. Some commentators have suggested that by rationing services, or by only having certain services available through the private sector, there will be an increase in efficiency. The previous chapter took pains to demonstrate that efficiency is not only about the costs and inputs side of the equation but about the relationship between inputs, on the one hand, and outputs and outcomes on the other. In other words, to achieve a measure of efficiency it is necessary to divert resources into those areas which secure the maximum benefit for the resources at society's disposal. What is rather unfortunate is that priority setting has become synonymous with rationing. It is the case that the term rationing has negative connotations, while establishing priorities has a more positive orientation, and does not necessarily involve cutting or reducing services, but rather attempts to ensure that resources are allocated efficiently by generating the maximum level of benefit for any given level of inputs. The current debate surrounding priorities in health care is characterised by considerable conflict, confusion and complexity (Coast and Donovan, 1996) and very little overall strategy as to how to address the problems of the health care dilemma.

A number of approaches have been employed to try and establish priorities in planning health care services (Donaldson, 1995; Mooney, 1994; Segal and Richardson, 1994) and they are outlined below:

History

The incremental approach adopted in budgets has led to many situations where one year's allocation of funds is carried forward to subsequent years with only minor adjustments made. However, no account is taken of whether one programme or 'budget-head' deserves a greater proportion of funding than other programmes or budget-heads because of differences in cost-effectiveness or the needs of the community. While this system may be administratively simplistic it does nothing to prioritise services to achieve improvements in the health of the population nor to enhance the efficiency of health care services.

Needs assessment and cost of illness studies

This is probably the most common approach employed to determine priorities and it has been argued that 'need has formed a basis for unacknowledged rationing within the NHS since its inception' (Frankel and West, 1993). The health care needs of communities or particular groups are assessed by surveys or epidemiological evidence, which provide an indication of the extent of ill health and disease and the implication for levels of morbidity, mortality and economic activity. Needs assessment provides the information on the dimension of health problems, priorities are then based on the size of the need and resources allocated in proportion to the diseases which have high mortality or morbidity rates. There are, however, a number of problems associated with needs assessment for determining priorities. The first surrounds the use of *total* needs. As Donaldson (1995) has argued, it is changes in need that are crucial. rather than the extent of the disease, and what can be done about it with the interventions available. Mooney (1994) is even more direct in his criticism, suggesting that 'needs assessment is based on faulty logic...(which) needs to be exposed and exposed again.' The second issue relates to the lack of consideration given to the costs of interventions or to the costs arising from policies designed to reduce the size of the problem. It is only by examining what costs are incurred in order to meet certain needs can any assessment be made of the efficiency of such interventions. In setting priorities it is therefore essential to be able to determine what is generated in terms of health improvements, reductions in mortality and what it costs to achieve these gains. Another point to note is that it is not necessary to assess the costs and benefits of all health care interventions. As has already been discussed the role of economics is to compare one allocation of resources with another. Thus, the question which should be posed is whether proposed changes will result in an improvement in the benefits for society over and above the current allocation of resources. This will be dealt with in more detail below, in the section dealing with programme budgeting and marginal analysis.

Target setting

This approach is a common feature of many health promotion policies where targets are specified and programmes are designed to reduce the incidence and prevalence of particular diseases. For example, the *Health of the Nation* identified key areas where a 'major' health problem existed...the Heartbeat Wales programme was established to reduce smoking prevalence by 5% over a five year period; the WHO set targets in their pursuit of the goal of Health for All by the Year 2000...; NHS hospitals are expected to meet a range of targets to comply with the Patients Charter....

However, as Segal and Richardson (1994) observed, 'with no formal method for assessing the capacity of health interventions to achieve nominated goals and targets, or the resource cost of achieving the objectives, the approach can provide little more than a 'wish list' of objectives.' Mooney (1994) examined the *Health of the Nation* targets and concluded that 'there is no consideration of costs; there is no consideration of the margin; there is no consideration of the benefits, except in rather a loose way; and there is no consideration of the weighing up of costs and benefits on the margin. It is sloganising for health in the sense of saying: let's get rid of the big health problems; rather than: let's maximise the health of the nation.' Not unsurprisingly, such an approach will not lead to allocative efficiency, a feature which according to Mooney (1994) is an opportunity missed 'to lead planners down the road of effective purchasing.'

Clinical guidelines/evidence based approaches

Clinical guidelines are the product of clinical groups gathered together as a Consensus Conference. They are used to inform clinical practice and can be a valuable part of the information base for making clinical decisions, while evidence-based medicine has been defined as 'the conscientious, explicit and

15

judicious use of current best evidence in making decisions about the care of individual patients' (Sackett et al., 1996). These approaches are critical in the move to ensure that services provided are clinically effective. It has been estimated, for example, that up to 25% of all health services currently provided may be unnecessary (Borowitz and Sheldon, 1993) and it has been illustrated that while 10-15% of health care interventions are known to generate health gain, a similar percentage are known to reduce health status. In the grey area are interventions whose effectiveness is either promising or have uncertain effects associated with them (Warner and Evans, 1993). Such approaches are vital in seeking to eradicate those interventions which are not effective in securing improvements in the health of the population. However, they cannot be expected to achieve allocative efficiency, as the process of drawing up clinical guidelines and arriving at a body of evidence does not incorporate a formal approach to the consideration of trade-offs between the costs and benefits of alternative options.

In fact, none of these approaches fit the requirements for achieving allocative efficiency and pay scant regard to the principles surrounding economics of competing demands for scarce resources. Two approaches which do fulfil the criteria are economic evaluation and programme budgeting and marginal analysis.

Economic evaluation

Economic evaluation involves assessing the volume of outputs and outcomes in relation to the level of inputs so as to arrive at an indicator of the relative efficiency of a project or programme. The important feature to note is that economic evaluation is concerned both with the costs incurred (the inputs) and the benefits generated (the outputs and outcomes). More detailed attention will be focused on economic evaluation in the next chapter, but in establishing a framework for priority setting economic evaluation does provide a useful departure point.

There are four techniques for undertaking economic evaluation but only two of them are of relevance in setting priorities. Cost minimisation and cost-effectiveness analysis are only able to deal with issues of technical efficiency but for allocative efficiency it is necessary to utilise cost-benefit (CBA) or cost-utility analysis (CUA). These two techniques aim to express health care outputs and outcomes in terms of monetary values (CBA) or in terms of utility (CUA) usually specified as Quality Adjusted Life Years (QALYs). Using CBA to evaluate the efficiency of options in order to establish priorities can be rather contentious, because the outcomes are measured in monetary terms and are therefore based on ability-to-pay. Therefore, there would appear to be an in-built bias in favour of those who are in employment, who enjoy relatively high income levels, the wealthy, etc. and a bias against the aged, the infirm, those with disabilities, those in poverty, the unemployed and so on.

The inherent dangers in using CBA have thus resulted in attention being focused on alternative ways of expressing the outputs and outcomes of health care interventions, based on specific disease-based measures of health status or on more generic indicators of quality of life. It is not the intention to review the literature here as there are a number of ideal reference sources to which the interested reader could turn (for example, Brooks, 1995; Bowling, 1995; Bowling, 1991; Hopkins, 1992; Hopkins, 1990; Johanesson et al., 1996; Wilkin, 1992). The use of CUA for establishing priorities is also controversial for a variety of theoretical and methodological reasons (Coast, 1996), but does provide a basis for comparisons across health care interventions. The approach of CUA is to estimate the costs associated with a particular intervention and its impact on both quantity and quality of life (Williams, 1985). From such studies it is possible, theoretically at least, to compare what is generated if £1 is spent in one area of health care as opposed to another area. For example, it has been shown that it cost £176 to generate one QALY if the resources were allocated to a cholesterol-lowering diet programme compared to £19,000 to yield one QALY in hospital haemodialysis for kidney failure (Ovretveit, 1995). However, there are a number of difficulties involved in the construction of such priority tables (Mason et al., 1993) to which further attention will be devoted in the next chapter. One of the major difficulties with 'explicit rational procedures' for establishing priorities is that they are 'vulnerable to subversion and highly costly' (Hunter, 1993) due to their vast data requirements. A more pragmatic approach has been advocated by other economists (Mooney et al., 1992), which recognises the difficulties associated with change. This is based on the techniques of marginal analysis and programme budgeting.

Programme budgeting and marginal analysis

Programme budgeting focuses on the outputs and outcomes of services in relation to the inputs used to generate such outputs and outcomes. The critical difference between programme budgeting and other types of budgeting rests in the emphasis given to the relationship between inputs and outputs/outcomes rather than concentrating on the inputs required. Programme budgeting, on its own, would not be a suitable technique for determining priorities. However, the incorporation of marginal analysis alongside programme budgeting does provide a 'framework to explore ways of improving the technical efficiency of programmes by examining the cost-effectiveness of the mix of inputs' (Posnett and Street, 1996). The concept of the margin is extremely important in economics. It focuses on the additional unit of a service and the cost of producing that particular unit and the benefits generated by that unit. It is thus possible to determine the extent of resources

17

to be allocated to a variety of different programmes and ensure that the benefits generated cannot be exceeded. This is when the ratio of marginal benefit to marginal cost is the same across all programmes. If the ratio of marginal benefit to marginal cost is 4:1 in Programme A and 2:1 in Programme B, a reallocation of resources from Programme B to Programme A would result in a net increase in benefits generated by both programmes. However, if both programmes had a ratio of 3:1 a reallocation of resources from one programme to the other would mean a net decrease in benefits. Maximum benefit will be achieved when the ratio of marginal benefit (MB) to marginal cost (MC) is the same across all programmes or sub-programmes, i.e. when:

$$\frac{MB_a}{MC_a} = \frac{MB_b}{MC_b} = \ldots\ldots\ldots\ldots\ldots\ldots \frac{MB_n}{MC_n}$$

There are a number of examples of where programme budgeting and marginal analysis have been employed (Cohen, 1994a; Craig et al., 1995; Twaddle and Walker, 1995). The basic approach of programme budgeting and marginal analysis (PBMA) has been outlined by Donaldson (1995). It involves four or five stages. The first stage is to identify the nature and constitution of a programme. Donaldson (1995) suggests that it may be more appropriate to actually start within programmes given that the paucity of outcome measures does not permit inter-programme comparisons, and hence have as Stage 1 the components of a programme, which can then be more clearly determined at Stage 2. This can be defined in terms of a disease group, such as asthma or diabetes, or by client group - the elderly or people with learning difficulties, for example. There are no hard and fast rules as to what actually constitutes a programme other than it must be output or outcome orientated and preferably disaggregated into sub-programmes.

The third stage involves setting out the expenditure on each programme and sub-programme and what is being generated by them. The means of identifying what is generated depends on the availability of information relating to outputs and outcomes. There is a great need for research to advance the relevance of output and outcome measures from the number of discharges or number of consultations to indicators which provide information relating to the actual impact on individuals' health. Despite the limitations of output and outcome information, this stage helps to define a programme and sub-programmes and enables a view to be taken of the expenditures incurred and outputs yielded before any consideration if given to the implications of moving resources.

The fourth stage is deciding which programmes and sub-programmes should receive an increase or a reduction in the resources allocated to them. By examining expenditure and activity on a particular sub-programme the view may be taken that it receives too much viz-a-viz other sub-programmes and might be a candidate for a potential reduction in resources. Conversely, other sub-programmes might be viewed in the opposite light and become entitled to an increase in resources.

The fifth stage is where the impact of proposed changes takes place, where marginal analysis has a role to play. Representatives of programmes and sub-programmes, the *expert group*, are asked how they would spend additional resources and what would be the effects on services and the health of the population, or, on the other hand, what services would be cut if resources were reduced and what would be the implications for health care within the area. The process revolves around these issues which examine, in the case of an increase in resources being made available, on which programme(s) or sub-programme(s) are they best spent in order to generate improvements in health: in the case of a reduction in resources, which programme(s) or sub-programme(s) should be cut to minimise the reductions in benefit; and, in the case of resources remaining constant, would a reallocation of resources from one programme or sub-programme to another result in an increase in total health care benefit?

It is not advocated however, that PBMA is problem free and a number of problems have been highlighted. For example, the time and information requirements may well prove to be a major constraint in undertaking a PBMA; the need to have a multi-disciplinary approach to PBMA compounds the time problem and the results of the exercise may be highly dependent upon the composition of the expert group (Posnett and Street, 1996); the asymmetry of information between providers and purchasers may result in possible contention in determining when to involve providers in the PBMA process, which can also result in excessive reliance on the literature on the part of purchasers (Donaldson, 1995); the lack of good quality data on outcomes forces the use of intermediate outputs, the maximisation of which may have detrimental effects elsewhere, as, for example, seeking to maximise consultant episodes may result in patients being discharged too early (Coast, 1996); and, PBMA may produce findings which are too broad to be of any practical value.

The role of the expert group in deciding which areas should be considered in the analysis has led 'to an inconsistency in applying the rigour of economic evaluations to options that have been selected in a way that is essentially arbitrary' and that the results of economic evaluations may be biased 'if the range of options selected for evaluation excludes viable alternatives' (Posnett and Street, 1996) They propose a flow diagram approach which maps

19

potential patient flows through the health care system and which identifies decision points where alternative service options are (or may be) available. The role of the expert group is thus concentrated on developing the flow diagram and highlighting sources of data rather than indicating the areas they wish to see considered in the analysis. This, they suggest removes the use of PBMA as a bargaining exercise and enhance its capability as a means of evaluating the resource and outcome consequences of all relevant options.

However, despite its limitations a number of PBMA studies have been undertaken with varying degrees of success. Cohen (1995) firmly believes that the criticisms should be kept in perspective and viewed as a means of securing improvements in the process. He concludes that 'application of the marginal analysis framework appears to offer a clear improvement in the way priorities are set.'

The technical problems surrounding economic approaches to priority setting should not be allowed to detract from the fact that they provide a rational framework within which other issues, such as considerations of equity and public and professional opinion, can be embraced and priorities established. According to Maynard (1994) 'these crude attempts to set priorities should be welcomed as a challenge to the covert, imprecise and inconsistent practice of prioritisation which exist in all health care systems today.'

The next chapter explores the techniques of economic evaluation in more detail prior to an investigation of how economic evaluation has been used in areas of health promotion activity. The final chapter reflects on how health promotion strategies may be guided by policies which are based on a set of priorities, based on a relatively systematic and scientific basis, as advocated by Normand (1994).

4. Economic evaluation

As indicated in Chapter 2, economic evaluation involves assessing the volume of outputs and outcomes in relation to the level of inputs so as to arrive at an indicator of the relative efficiency of a project or programme. It has been defined as 'a comparative analysis of two or more alternatives in terms of their costs and consequences' (Kobelt, 1996).There is an abundance of sources within the literature which explain and apply the principles of economic evaluation (for example, Drummond et al., 1987; Kobelt, 1996; McGuire, 1988) and also a number which provide general applications in health promotion and related fields (for example, Barry and DeFriese, 1990; Cohen, 1992; Cohen, 1994b; Cohen and Henderson, 1988; Tolley, 1993).

This chapter has four distinct phases. The first phase considers the framework of economic evaluation; the second phase explains the techniques of economic evaluation; the third phase considers some of the methodological issues surrounding economic evaluation and health promotion; and, the fourth phase highlights the approach adopted in reviewing the impact of economic evaluation in health promotion.

The framework of economic evaluation

The framework for economic evaluation can be depicted as shown in the diagram, figure 4.1 on p.22.

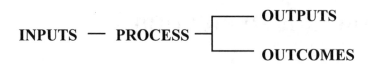

Figure 4.1: The economic evaluation framework

The terms inputs, processes, outputs and outcomes have been defined as follows: inputs - resources invested in specified official activities; processes - a series of actions and interactions; outputs - measurable product(s) attributable to an input or combination of inputs; outcomes - end-state(s) which may or may not be the intended effect of specified inputs, outputs or processes (Phillips et al., 1994). A more pertinent set of definitions relevant for health promotion have been developed based on a model of performance indicators (Whelan et al., 1993). The role of performance indicators in health promotion have been discussed and refined further by Buck et al. (1996) and it appears that much research remains to be done before a clear set of indicators can be arrived at. However, this remains true of outcome determination and measurement in general in health care. While recognising the limitations of the current state of the art it need not prevent attempts to evaluate the efficiency of health promotion programmes and other areas of health care from taking place. The role of economics within such an evaluation framework is to consider the relationship between inputs, processes, outputs and outcomes to assess whether outputs and outcomes are maximised given the level of inputs or whether the level of inputs are minimised given the levels of outputs and outcomes.

The importance attached to economic evaluations by policy makers, planners and managers has been evidenced by the growth in the literature of economic evaluations in health care. Accompanying this growth, have been studies which have attempted to assess the contribution of such evaluations to the decision making process (Drummond et al., 1996; Luce, 1996) and initiatives designed to develop systems of good practice and adopt a standardised approach to economic evaluation (see for example, Gerard, 1992; Drummond et al., 1987 ; Drummond et al., 1993a; Johannesson et al., 1996; Luce and Elixhauser, 1990; Phillips et al., 1994).

There are six distinct phases in undertaking an economic evaluation, each of which need to be present if the study is to conform to the guidelines of good practice. The six phases are:

- The description of the policy under which the project is being considered, alternative ways of achieving the policy goals, and the specification of the objectives for each of the alternative approaches.

- The identification of all relevant costs and benefits associated with the project and its alternatives.

- The measurement and valuation of the relevant costs and benefits.

- The comparison between the costs and benefits, having adjusted for the effects of time and uncertainty and the choice of discount rate to employ.

- The decision criteria with which to identify the most 'efficient' alternative.

- The carrying out of a sensitivity analysis on the findings.

Each of the phases will now be considered and suggestions made as to how to undertake each stage, pointing out some of the potential problems and how they may be overcome.

The description of the policy, alternatives of implementation and specification of objectives

Until this initial stage has been undertaken adequately the subsequent stages have no foundation. The policy to be evaluated must be clearly described and the alternative ways of implementing it considered for the evaluator to have a clear perspective on which to construct the investigation. For example, consider the situation where the government has initiated a policy designed to reduce the incidence of heart disease within the country. There are a number of possible ways of tackling the problem. Central government could intervene directly and levy additional taxation on smoking. Alternatively it could provide extra resources to the health authorities to commission a series of health promotion programmes or to employ additional health education officers, who could then implement local strategies to reduce the scale of the problem. In this situation the evaluator would have to be aware of the policy (the reduction of heart disease), the alternatives (as identified above in part) and the objectives of each of the alternative ways of implementing the policy. In deciding which technique to utilise the evaluator needs to be aware of whether there is a fixed benefit or effect to be achieved (e.g. reduction in smoking prevalence by x%), and hence use *cost-effectiveness analysis*, whether the objective is to increase *quality adjusted life years* and use *cost-utility analysis*, or whether the objective is to ensure that the net social gain in monetary terms (e.g. the impact on gross national product of a decline in premature deaths and absenteeism associated

23

with heart disease as compared with the costs of implementing the policy) is maximised and hence use *cost-benefit analysis*.

The identification of all relevant costs and benefits

The use of economic evaluation requires that all costs and benefits are identified, i.e. that both private and social costs and benefits need to be included. For example, the true costs of community care include the costs to the agencies for providing the particular packages of care plus the costs to individuals and society of providing informal care to the elderly and disabled within their communities. The importance of this particular stage cannot be over-emphasised. Even though it may not be possible to measure and value all costs and benefits, all relevant costs and benefits associated with the policy must be identified so that the decision-maker is fully aware of *all* of the consequences of the actions undertaken. In other words the difficulties of quantification and valuation should not preclude the existence of all costs and benefits from the 'balance sheet' of costs and benefits to be considered by the decision-maker. In some situations there may be a case for categorising the costs and benefits into those which impact on the 'public purse' and those which have wider social implications. An example of such an approach is to be found in Phillips and Prowle (1993), where the authors identify, measure and value the costs and benefits of Heartbeat Wales No-Smoking Intervention Programme from the viewpoint of the Exchequer and also from society as a whole.

Whether or not all costs and benefits are identified, the results of any evaluation should be subjected to a sensitivity analysis, where those costs and benefits which have not been measured and/or valued should be re-introduced in order to examine the reliability and accuracy of the findings. For example, if a project demonstrates a small net loss overall *but* only one or two of a long list of benefits have been measured and valued there is scope for speculation that if more of the benefits had been included in the calculations then the project might have shown a net overall gain.

The measurement and valuation of costs

When measuring the costs of a policy it must be remembered that resources utilised in one area cannot be used in another, that is a cost is always a foregone benefit. This notion of *opportunity cost* was introduced in chapter 2 and can be defined as 'the satisfaction that would have been gained from pursuing the next best alternative activity on a preference listing.' In many cases the price that a person pays for a good in the market reflects its opportunity cost and the pragmatic approach to costing in economic evaluation is to take the existing market price wherever possible.

In situations where market prices are not appropriate (because, for example, they fail to consider externalities) or where they are not available, the evaluator may adopt the concept of *shadow prices*, which has been defined as 'the price the economist attributes to a good or factor on the argument that it is more appropriate for the purpose of economic calculation than its existing price, if any' (Mishan, 1982). For example, clean-air may be valued by the premium people are prepared to pay for houses in a 'clean-air zone.'

Another important concept in the economist's repertoire is that of 'marginal cost.' The marginal cost is the cost associated with one additional unit of product, activity or service. As discussed in Chapter 3, the concept of the margin is extremely important in the context of setting priorities and in policy evaluation, because in many cases the alternatives will not necessarily be whether a particular service is to be provided or not, but whether the size of a service should be expanded or reduced. In such cases, the costs measured should be the cost of increasing (or reducing) the service, that is the marginal cost. For example, the additional cost of extending the provision of a mobile screening service for breast cancer to a new estate in an urban area is relatively small compared to the additional cost of providing the same service to a new house in a remote rural area. Problems arise in evaluation when average, rather than marginal. costs are used since they fail to allow for variations in intensity of current resource utilisation.

Another aspect of cost measurement and valuation that needs to be carefully considered is the treatment of *capital costs*. These costs are incurred when the major assets of the programme are acquired, i.e. the buildings, the equipment, etc. Capital costs are not merely the sum actually paid for their acquisition and the interest payments on any loans used to fund such purchases. Account also has to be taken of the opportunity cost of using such assets in one particular way, thereby depriving them from being used elsewhere. For example, long after the land, buildings and equipment have been paid for, there is a capital cost of continuing to use the facilities as long as it could be used in an alternative way.

A further difficulty arises in the area of costs which are not unique to the project in question. For example, a hospital in-patient receives treatment which involves inputs of medical staff, other staff, drugs, dressings, diagnostic tests, etc. but the hospital also incurs other costs in the form of maintenance of grounds and equipment, general management, cleaning and so on, which are reflected in the overall costs of the hospital. However, if the system of marginal costs and marginal benefits is adhered to the evaluation need only consider the additional resources required to treat the patient, or alternatively, what resources will be released for the use of others.

25

The measurement and valuation of benefits can be an involved and complicated process. The nature of benefits in health care and health promotion in particular are subject to much debate and consideration. The stream of benefits flowing from a health care intervention can be classified into three types as shown in the diagram, figure 4.2, below:

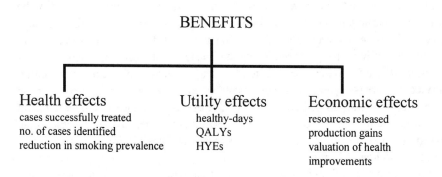

BENEFITS

Health effects
cases successfully treated
no. of cases identified
reduction in smoking prevalence

Utility effects
healthy-days
QALYs
HYEs

Economic effects
resources released
production gains
valuation of health
improvements

Figure 4.2 The benefits of a health care intervention

The whole issue of identifying, measuring and valuing benefits determines the type of economic evaluation which can be undertaken. When the outcomes are measured in terms of health effects the technique to employ is cost effectiveness analysis; when the outcomes are measured in terms of utility effects the approach is to use cost utility analysis; when the outcomes are measured in terms of economic (monetary) effects the technique to employ is that of cost benefit analysis. If the outcomes from two or more alternative programmes are identical the approach is cost minimisation because in these circumstances it is only the difference in costs which needs to be considered. More attention will be devoted to these techniques in the next section of the chapter and more discussion on the issues surrounding outcome measurement in health promotion is contained in the third section of this chapter.

Given most people's preferences for *current* consumption rather than *potential future* consumption, the costs and benefits which occur at the present time must be valued more highly than those which accrue in the future. In order to allow for this future costs and benefits are subjected to *discounting*, which brings *all* costs and benefits to the present time. The approach is quite simple. If we expect to receive a benefit of £10,000 in five years time, the present value of that, based on a discount rate of 5%, is equivalent to £7,835. The approach is to multiply the benefit by a discount factor based on the discount rate chosen:

Year	Benefit	Discount factor	Present value
1	10,000	0.9524	9,524
2	10,000	0.9070	9,070
3	10,000	0.8638	8,638
4	10,000	0.8227	8,227
5	10,000	0.7835	7,835

The difficulty in health care arises in determining whether or not to discount health gains in the future and, if so, at which rate of interest to employ in discounting future costs and benefits. This issue will be further discussed later in section 3 of the chapter.

Basically, there are two approaches to adopt in selecting which discount rate to employ in weighting future costs and benefits. The former involves the social time preference (STP) rate and the latter the social opportunity cost of capital (SOC). The STP is based on individuals' time preferences whilst the SOC reflects the opportunity cost of postponement of receipt of any benefit emerging from the implementation, of a programme involving public funds. However, the practical choice of which rate to choose is complicated by the presence of externalities, uncertainty and the lack of any clear perception of what might constitute the time preference rate of society. Obviously, the choice of a discount rate will have a significant impact upon the relative value of a project but as yet no consensus has emerged as to the correct rate to use. In practice, most public projects utilise the official test discount rate recommended by the Treasury as being the SOC rate, it being the marginal rate of return on private sector investment and thus represents the opportunity cost of public sector investment, although there have been suggestions that reliance on the SOC fails to incorporate equity judgements as would be the case if the STP were used. Therefore, wherever possible a compromise rate is chosen and sensitivity analysis utilised to determine the impact of changes in the rate on the findings of the evaluation.

One of the major reasons why people prefer current rather than future consumption is the fact that we live in a world of uncertainty - nothing is guaranteed, other than death. Therefore, it cannot safely be assumed that the programme will definitely result in certain outputs and outcomes. The use of sensitivity analysis is the usual approach to adopt in allowing for uncertainty. However, some other methods have been offered in the literature, (see for example, Pearce and Nash, 1981; Mishan, 1983; Dasgupta and Pearce, 1974), which range from the concept of *risk aversion* through *game-theory*, where *maximin and minimax* strategies are used, to the use of *probability factors*, where potential outcomes are weighted by factors which represent the likelihood of such events occurring. Given the problems associated with such methods, the general approach is to ensure that an adequate sensitivity analysis is incorporated as an integral part of the economic evaluation.

Decision criteria

In principle there are a number of potential methods for assessing the worth of a range of alternatives:

1. Cut-off period: A suitable period is chosen over which the costs incurred must be fully recouped. This may be because of the considerable uncertainty surrounding the benefits occurring in the future. However, the danger of such a method is that projects whose benefits do not materialise to any great extent until some time in the future would be disregarded, e.g. the outcomes associated with a health promotion programme may not accrue for a considerable period of time. Despite the fact that such benefits offset the costs incurred many times over, the project would fail to be allocated resources if the cut-off period method were employed.

2. Pay-off period: Instead of choosing an arbitrary cut-off period, the alternatives may be ranked according to the number of years necessary to recoup the initial outlay. It may be that in conditions of extreme political uncertainty, where safety is one of the overriding considerations, such an approach may be appropriate. However, this method suffers from the same limitations as the cut-off period and as a result in often used alongside one of the methods which takes account of the time factor, that is the Net Present Value and Internal Rate of Return methods (see, for example, Phillips and Prowle, 1993).

3. Average rate of return: This method simply aggregates the benefits associated with the project, divides the sum by the number of years over which the benefits accrue and expresses the result as a percentage of the initial outlay. However, on this basis a project which has a return of £1,000 in the first year only would have a greater rate of return than one, with the same initial outlay, which achieved returns of £500 per year for five years. Another difficulty with this method is that no account is taken of the profile of benefits, i.e. a project which has benefits of £200, £400, £600, £800 in years 1 to 4 would have exactly the same rate of return as a project with benefits of £800, £600, £400 and £200 in years 1 to 4. In other words the effect of time on the value of future benefits is not considered at all in the method.

4. Net Present Value (NPV): The NPV of a project is the sum of the benefits accruing during the project's lifetime less the present value of costs. As opposed to the methods referred to above the NPV approach does recognise that the timing of the costs and flow of benefits can be extremely important in determining the 'best' alternative. In deciding between alternatives the NPV approach would be to select the project with the greatest NPV, subject to a sensitivity analysis which adjusts for any uncertainties involved.

5. The Internal Rate of Return (IRR): The IRR is another method which takes account of the effects of time. The IRR is basically the discount rate which equates the present value of all the benefits with the present value of all the costs, that is the IRR is the discount rate for which the NPV is equal to zero. For example, if a project which costs £150,000 has benefits of £40,000 for each of four years then the IRR would be 10.4%, since the present value of £40,000 over four years is £150,000 at a discount rate of 10.4%.

Sensitivity analysis

It will be clear from the discussion so far that economic evaluation is not an exact science. There are many issues which point to the need to treat the findings of such evaluations with considerable caution. It is therefore essential that in undertaking an economic evaluation of a health promotion programme a sensitivity analysis should be incorporated. As the term implies the approach is to test how sensitive the results obtained are by considering 'what if' type scenarios and questions. In other words the effects of changes in the costs incurred, the benefits accruing from the projects and the discount rate will all have to be examined before the results of the evaluation can be delivered to the relevant decision maker(s). An example of this approach was used by Phillips and Prowle (1993) in assessing the impact of a No-Smoking intervention. The initial results were tested to examine the impact of three alternative scenarios:

firstly, if the benefits had been 10% or 20% less; secondly, if there had been a 5 year delay in receiving the benefits; and thirdly, if there had been a 5 year delay and the benefits were 10% less.

The techniques of economic evaluation

Under the umbrella of economic evaluation there are four techniques available, depending on how the consequences of health care interventions and programmes are measured and valued. These techniques are described in detail elsewhere (see for example, Brooks, 1995; Cohen, 1992; Kobelt, 1996). However, it is worth providing a brief overview of the techniques in order to appreciate some of the issues discussed in chapters five to twelve.

Cost minimisation analysis

Where the outcomes of two or more programmes are identical. or vary only slightly, and there is no significant difference in the effectiveness, then the choice between programmes in terms of efficiency would be made on the basis of costs with the less costly alternative being the preferred choice.

Cost effectiveness analysis

In the large majority of cases there will probably be differing degrees of success in achieving outcomes as well as differences in costs. The choice is then made on the basis of *cost per unit of effect* or *effects per unit of cost* with the programme with the least cost per unit of effect (or greatest effects per unit of cost) being the most efficient. Tolley (1993), for example, illustrated how cost effectiveness analysis would be used to distinguish between programmes designed to reduce the incidence of smoking by comparing the *cost per quitter* resulting from the UK National No-Smoking Day and a national mass media campaign. Using data from Reid et al. (1992) the cost per quitter from the No-Smoking Day was approximately £20 (1992 prices) compared to approximately £13 per quitter from the mass media campaign. Tolley (1993) stated that 'the no-smoking day is less cost-effective than the national media campaign.' He also introduced an extremely important caveat at this juncture by indicating that 'for health promotion managers with cash limited budgets this evidence may not provide much useful guidance for decision making' since the benefits from the mass media campaign are contingent upon a much larger investment of funds. In order to deduce whether the additional resources needed to finance the media campaign would be worthwhile there is need to place a monetary value on the benefits generated by each of the

30

alternative programmes so as to assess which has the greatest cost-benefit ratio. This is the basis of cost benefit analysis, which is discussed below.

There are two stages to cost-effectiveness analysis: the first stage involves arriving at the average and marginal costs and effects of the interventions, often using techniques such as decision analysis (Weinstein, 1990) and Markov analysis (Sonneberg and Beck, 1993). The second stage is to calculate and compare the cost-effectiveness ratios for each of the alternatives, with the important indicator being the *incremental cost-effectiveness ratio*, which shows the cost of generating an extra unit of effect.

Cost benefit analysis

In most instances it is unlikely that the outcomes of programmes are identical. Indeed, comparison may need to be made between two completely diverse programmes where the outcomes are entirely different. In order to assess the relative efficiency the outcomes would have to be translated into a common denominator, usually a monetary measure, and the results stated in either the form of a ratio of costs and benefits, expressed in money terms, or as a sum representing the net benefit (or loss) of one programme over another. For example, the savings generated to the health service and employers by people not contracting coronary heart disease because of improved dietary intake could be compared with the savings generated by the closure of long stay mental hospitals.

Cost benefit analysis enables the notion of efficiency to be viewed from a higher level, that of *allocative efficiency*, in that it enables judgements to be made about the relative value of pursuing one objective (reduction in CHD) as opposed to another (emphasis on community care). Cost effectiveness analysis, on the other hand, can only provide an indication of *technical efficiency*, since it provides an assessment of different ways of fulfilling the same objective (for example, reducing smoking prevalence).

However, cost benefit analysis is reliant on being able to place monetary values on the identified costs and benefits. This is possible where market prices exist, or when shadow prices can be used as proxies, for example, what people are willing to pay for reduced risks. Methods of arriving at indicators of willingness-to-pay can be arrived at by asking people directly through, for example, questionnaires. One such method is the *contingent valuation approach*, which asks people the maximum amount they would be prepared to pay for the benefit. An alternative to the questionnaire approach is to employ proxy values, for example, the price people are prepared to pay for receiving treatment in a private hospital would be an indicator of how much they were willing to pay to avoid having to join a waiting list.

31

The major issue confronting any cost benefit analysis is what value can be placed on human life? If contribution to production is used as the imputed value then this would mean that the elderly, people with learning difficulties and others who make no contribution to the economy would be assigned a zero value! Who is to determine the value of human life? Willingness-to-pay is but one approach, which according to Cohen (1992) 'is conceptually pleasing because it attempts to tease out the values of those actually at risk' but also 'can be criticised on several grounds.' For a fuller discussion of the concept see, for example, Donaldson et al.,1995; O'Brien and Viramaster, 1994; Mooney and Lange, 1993; Thompson, 1986; Johannesson and Jonsson, 1991. Other methods on valuing benefits rely on estimates made by practitioners, professionals and policy-makers, for example, the compensation paid by a court to offset the consequences of medical negligence could be used in the valuation process.

Cost utility analysis

An alternative measure of value to that of a monetary approach is one of utility. This sort of analysis considers the impact of the policy upon an individual's and society's welfare, expressed in some quantitative measure. This approach, which can be used to judge both technical efficiency and allocative efficiency (Gerard, 1992), is being increasingly used in the evaluation of health-care policies where *quality of life* adjustments are made to a given state of outcomes, whilst simultaneously providing a common denominator for comparison of costs and outcomes in different health-care programmes. The common denominator, usually expressed *as healthy days, well-years* (Kaplan, 1988), *quality adjusted life years* (QALYs) or *healthy years equivalent* (HYEs) is arrived at by adjusting the duration of the outcome (e.g. life expectancy) by the utility value of the resulting health status. For a discussion of the relative merits of which denominator to employ see Johannesson et al. (1996).

The basis of using utility effects is based on the notion that outcomes from treatments and other health influencing activities have two basic components, quantity and quality of life. Life expectancy is a traditional measure with few problems of comparison. However, attempts to measure and value quality of life have a more recent history, with a number of approaches and instruments being utilised. Particular effort has gone into researching ways in which an overall health index might be constructed which would locate a specific health state on a continuum between, for example, 0 (= death) and 1 (= perfect health). Obviously, the portrayal of health in this way is far removed from an ideal representation since, for example, the definition of perfect health is highly subjective while it has also been argued that some health states are worse than death.

The construction of such measures has a number of possible uses, for example, in to identify public health trends to enable strategies to be developed; to assess the effectiveness and efficiency of health care interventions; and, to determine the state of health in communities.

The Quality Adjusted Life Year (QALY) has been created to combine the quantity and quality of life. The basic idea of a QALY is straightforward. It takes one year of perfect-health life expectancy to be worth 1, but regards one year of less than perfect-health life expectancy as less than 1. Thus, an intervention which results in a patient living for an additional four years, rather than dying within a year, but where the quality of life falls from 1 (perfect-health) to 0.6 on the continuum, will generate :

4 years extra life @ 0.6 quality of life value = 2.4
less 1 year @ reduced quality (i.e. 1 - 0.6) = 0.4

QALYs generated by intervention = 2.0

QALYs can thus provide an indication of the benefits gained from a variety of medical procedures, in terms of quality of life and survival for the patient. For a fuller explanation of how to arrive at QALYs the reader is referred to Johannesson et al. (1996), Williams (1995), Kobelt (1996).

It is no use in pretending that QALYs are anything but a crude measurement of both survival and quality of life as they currently stand. It is necessary, therefore, to be aware of their limitations and hope that further research can improve the concept making it more sophisticated. However, the use of QALYs in resource allocation decisions does mean that choices between patient groups competing for medical care are made explicit. QALYs have been criticised because there is an implication that some patients will be refused or not offered treatment for the sake of other patients and, yet, such choices have been made and are being made all the time. Even if the NHS were allocated a considerable increase in resources it would still be necessary to make choices.

The question needs to be asked on what basis are these choices and priorities being made? Are the decisions equally fair to all patient groups? Are there any patient groups who consistently receive less or poorer health care, or who consistently suffer poor health? As members of society, doctors and nurses have a responsibility to society as a whole and not only to individual patients, despite the fact than when faced with an ill patient it is painful to realise that treatment of this patient may be at the expense of another.

It should be the case that the choices made are the efficient and humane ones, and not merely based on political pressures or the quest for technological advancement. There is a clear need for a constituency wider than the medical profession itself in assessing treatment priorities. To restrict decision making to doctors, or for that matter administrators, is to allow the continuance of the current system of resource allocation where most resources go to those who shout the loudest or to those who pluck the heartstrings the hardest. Widening the decision making process is a move in the direction of ensuring a more humane system and the utilisation of QALYs (despite their limitations) is a means whereby the outputs generated by the health care system can be included in the process, thereby enabling decisions to be made which will maximise the benefits of health care provision for society.

The development of QALYs (and its close relations) has also led to the production of QALY league tables (for example, Williams, 1985; Maynard, 1991). One of the noticeable features of these tables is that health promotion programmes and other preventive measures are located towards the top end of the table, and as Drummond (1992a) implies that 'interventions near the top of the list are better value for money than those at the bottom,' it would appear that some health promotion schemes can be viewed as being relatively efficient. For example, the cost of generating a QALY via a programme of cholesterol testing and diet therapy for adults aged 40-69 is £220 and GP advice to stop smoking is £270 per QALY compared to £7,840 for heart transplantation and £107,780 for neurosurgical intervention for malignant intracranial tumours. However, there are some preventive schemes which perform less well in terms of cost/QALY indicators. Breast cancer screening costs £5,780 to generate a QALY while cholesterol testing and treatment (incrementally) for adults aged 25-39 costs £14,150. (All figures are in August 1990 prices and taken from Maynard, 1991)

The construction and use of QALY league tables has generated considerable discussion and debate (Drummond, 1989; Drummond et al., 1993; Gerard, 1992; Petrou et al., 1993). More specifically, there remain a number of questions about the appropriateness of QALYs for measuring the outcomes of health promotion. Cribb and Haycox (1989) have argued that they are too insensitive for evaluating the effectiveness of health promotion. They argue that this is due to their inclusion of a large and indeterminate number of variables, the lower reliability of the perceived values generated and an inability to allow for the longer term effects of cumulative health improvements resulting from changes in behaviour and lifestyle. The use of a 0-1 scale inevitably means that those individuals already high up the scale will not record significant actual health gains resulting from exposure to health promotion campaigns.

In summing up this section it is worth remembering that there is no 'gold standard' or 'best' QOL measure, and it is probably best not to think in such terms. QOL is a subjective and fluid-end point, so its measurement must include the patient's perspective and be sensitive to change over time. In addition to the important theoretical and empirical elements of QOL measurement, practical issues such as timing or administration...are likely to provide obstacles to accurate measurement...It is important to be aware of the strengths and weaknesses of available measures when setting out to study quality of life' (Erickson et al. 1995).

Methodological issues surrounding economic evaluation and health promotion

Outcome measures

The cost utility approach, as with other approaches to economic evaluation, are somewhat flawed due to a number of methodological issues. Firstly, as indicated above, debate and discussion surrounds the nature of the outcome measures used in the analyses. Many studies have relied on mortality reduction, or variations on this theme (for example, avoidable life years (Godfrey et al., 1989), as an indicator of health promotion effectiveness. However, this is not very appropriate where interventions have a greater impact on morbidity or aspects relating to quality of life. Whereas, well-years and QALYs would enable the combination of mortality and morbidity factors there is also a case for distinguishing between the implications for mortality and the impact on morbidity from changes in behaviour relating to 'health-damaging' activities (Nutbeam et al., 1991).

Problems also arise from the exclusion of non-health related benefits. For example, there are the *consumption* benefits resulting from participation in exercise and from health education (Engleman and Forbes, 1986), the 'idea that individuals can receive peace of mind from the knowledge that their risk levels have been reduced' (Cohen and Henderson, 1988), while Rosen and Lindholm (1992) catalogued the benefits and risks not included in economic evaluations of health promotion and argued that the results obtained may bias the results and lead to a less than optimal use of available resources. They highlighted the neglect of considering factors such as changes in mortality and morbidity of 'other diseases,' changes in self-esteem due to attempts to change lifestyle, changes in consumption values due to lifestyle changes, changes in anxiety, economic incentives and social diffusion and also argued that they are not insignificant. There are also other aspects which would not be considered within the parameters of the economic evaluation. For example, successful intervention preventing the onset of one disease may result in greater probability of acquiring other diseases later in life (Schaapveld et al., 1990) and should be included in any estimate of life years gained.

All these issues surround the debate as to what should be regarded as the *final outcome measure* of health promotion. The nature of health promotion activities necessitate the use of *process indicators* and *intermediate outcomes* (Tolley, 1993; Whelan et al., 1993) or *indirect, intermediate, behavioural. subjective and clinical indicators* (Tones et al., 1991; Tones, 1992) which highlight the need for evaluations to utilise appropriate outcome measures bearing in mind the nature and scope of the programme, and its alternatives, under consideration.

Cost of illness studies

There is a substantial literature on cost of illness studies, and much work on prevention of illness draws on the results of such investigations, with the logic being that if health promotion activities can prevent such illnesses then the savings generated can be substantial. There is a fundamental issue at stake here in that health promotion should not be seen merely as a scheme for reducing health care costs, partly since there is much debate as to whether it does actually achieve this (for example, Leu and Schaub, 1983, 1985; Higgins, 1988; Fries et al., 1989; St. Leger, 1989; Godfrey, 1993) but more importantly, because health promotion activities can produce significant health gains in reducing premature death and improvements in quality of life but at a net cost. To quote Williams (1990):

> I even believe that being efficient is a *moral obligation*, not just a managerial convenience, for *not* to be efficient means imposing avoidable death and unnecessary suffering on people who might have benefited from the resources which are being used wastefully.

The role of economic evaluation is to seek to ensure that available resources are channeled into the most beneficial activities and therefore generate an efficient allocation of resources. However, the use of cost of illness studies as a basis for establishing priorities, according to Mooney (1994), 'will not lead to an efficient allocation of resources, nor is it a way of getting to something approximating to efficiency.' The discussion as to what should and what should not be included in cost of illness studies (Drummond, 1992b; Hodgson, 1994) is particularly relevant for any examination of the effectiveness of health promotion activities. Exclusion of indirect costs, for example, from cost of illness studies may well understate the extent to which health promotion activities can generate efficiencies. Drummond (1992b) also highlights the risk that policy makers may be misled into thinking that cost of illness studies give guidance on whether or not more resources should be devoted to a given disease and argues that 'these issues can only be addressed by considering the costs and effectiveness of interventions for the disease in question.' The implication for health promotion agencies is therefore apparent - the need to determine the most efficient ways of promoting health to maximise health gain in society rather than concentrating resources in activities to reduce prevalence in particular disease categories. As Cohen (1994) points out 'decisions in health care are rarely of the do or don't variety' but rather revolve around whether to alter the allocation of resources in favour of one scheme rather than an alternative.

Discounting

The issue of whether preventive health schemes are more cost-effective than curative schemes depends in part on how future health gains are valued. The theory of time preference states that, in general. people prefer present consumption to potential consumption sometime in the future, and therefore, health gains, costs and benefits, which accrue over time must be brought into line with costs and benefits which accrue at the present. The technique of discounting is employed to achieve this so that future flows of health care savings, improved quality of life, etc. are valued at current 'rates.' The method of discounting was discussed earlier, and the issue of whether health care benefits should be subjected to discounting and if so, what discount rate to employ was also referred to.

The magnitude of discount rate varies between 3% and 10% in the literature, and the current rate for use in the UK is the 6% official test discount rate recommended by the Treasury as being the social opportunity cost rate. This rate represents the marginal return on private sector investment and thus represents the opportunity cost of public sector investment. Drummond et al. (1993), while not advocating the same rate for all countries, do suggest that analysts would be willing to employ a 5% discount rate to assist in making comparisons among studies.

As to whether health care benefits should be discounted there appears to be a range of views. While there is a consensus that both costs and outcomes should be discounted at the appropriate rate when they are measured in monetary terms (Drummond et al., 1993), there is less consensus as to whether non-financial gains should be subjected to the same process. There are those who argue for consistency (for example, Katz and Welch, 1993; Williams, 1981), those who argue for a differential rate for health outcomes (for example, Goodin, 1982); those who argue for a zero, or virtually zero, rate (for example, West, 1996; Parsonage and Neuberger, 1992), which has

37

been recommended by the Department of Health for all new economic studies of health programmes; and, those who argue that it may be wise to present the benefits discounted in the base case analysis and with no discounting in the sensitivity analysis (Johannesson et al., 1996). Coyle and Tolley (1992) argued strongly against valuing future health benefits at a lower rate since to do so was unethical and based on invalid arguments in that decisions to smoke and drink may be related to a low perceive risk of ill health from such behaviour rather than a preference to indulge now and pay later, in terms of reduced health status.

The implications of a zero discount rate are particularly relevant for health promotion schemes which produce 'longer-term' benefits, since the differences between discounted and non-discounted benefit flows can be quite marked. For example, Parsonage and Neuberger (1992) demonstrated that the effect of employing a zero discount rate as opposed to a 6% rate would reduce the cost of generating a QALY (1990 prices) from nicotine gum for male smokers aged 35-39 would fall from £3,750 to £750.

Tolley (1993) has proposed two approaches which could be employed to address the problems associated with the timing of the costs and outcomes of a health promotion programme. Firstly, he suggests more attention being focused on the short-run benefits of health promotion, which would help to reduce the reliance on single outcome measures for comparing programmes and enable the consumption benefits of health promotion to be given increasing prominence. Adopting a slightly different approach (Nutbeam et al., 1991) estimated the payback period for the Heartbeat Wales No-Smoking intervention, arguing that 'it offers a useful tool for risk-averse investors who wish to see quick returns on their investments.' More appropriately, the approach would be useful for purchasers, who faced with current cases waiting for treatment, are being urged to commit resources to health promotion and preventive schemes, 'where the health gains are anonymous and way in the future' (Godfrey, 1993).

The second approach offered by Tolley (1993) is to utilise the sensitivity analysis to examine the effect of employing a series of discount rates on the flow of health benefits. This would, at least, enable deliberations to be focused on those areas where different valuations of future health care benefits are crucial. This is the approach advocated by Katz and Welch (1993), who argues that decision makers need to be aware of the biases introduced by discounting, for example, the lives of children would be valued higher than those of the elderly.

Is prevention more efficient than cure?

One area where valuation of future health care benefits are crucial is in relation to the issue of whether prevention (health promotion) is more efficient than cure. The issue has long been the subject of debate in the literature, although the emphasis has tended to be on whether health promotion can exert downward pressure on the utilisation of other health care facilities and on costs. It has been estimated that preventable illness constitutes approximately 70% of the burden of illness and the associated costs (Fries et al., 1993) and therefore the incentives to utilise health promotion and preventive measures for such a purpose are obviously attractive. However, there are two basic issues at stake! Firstly, is there evidence that prevention and health promotion do reduce health care costs and secondly, whether health promotion should be subjected to such an evaluative criterion?

With regard to the first issue it is probably the case that the 'jury is still out!' (Russell, 1986; Barry and DeFriese, 1990; Higgins, 1988; Pelletier, 1991; Lynch and Vickery, 1993; Shephard, 1987). The lack of irrefutable evidence for the effectiveness of prevention and/or health promotion in securing changes in mortality and morbidity, coupled with the dependency on securing reasonable participation rates in schemes, presents an obvious difficulty in arriving at a firm conclusion. Differentials in timing between programmes and their 'effects' compounds the difficulty, especially when future benefits are subject to discounting, and the question remains as to whether prolonging people's lives results in a postponement of their demands on health care resources (Leu and Schaub, 1983; Leu and Schaub, 1985; Fries et al., 1989; St. Leger, 1989; Nutbeam et al., 1991).

The second, and in some sense the more important, issue stems from the fact that other health care activities do not include 'impact on cost reduction' inserted within their evaluative framework. Health promotion deserves to be treated in the same way. It is agreed that health promotion, as an activity, is not costless to society - there are sacrifices and risks associated with participation. The question to be addressed is whether allocating resources to health promotion activities is going to provide a return to society in terms of improved health and reductions in disabilities and premature deaths. As with all areas, there will be some schemes that prove to be a waste of scarce resources, while others are highly efficient in securing large scale benefits from the resources invested.

A compromise or trade-off position between the 'cost reduction' and 'health gain' perspectives can be depicted by developing the notion of the *policy space* (Anderson, 1986; Kaplan, 1988) . This is shown in Figure 4.3. The horizontal axis measures the net benefits to the health service and/or

39

society expressed in monetary terms while the vertical axis measures the net health gain achieved by the programme:

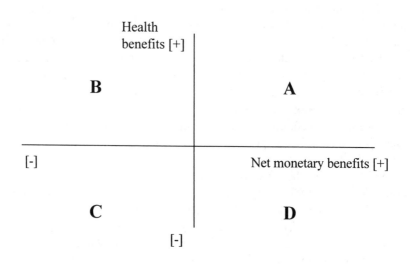

Figure 4.3: The health policy space (adapted from Anderson, 1986 and Kaplan, 1988)

Therefore, programmes in Quadrant A would demonstrate both net benefits to society (that is, a reduction in overall costs) plus improvements in health status, represented by mortality and morbidity reduction; programmes in Quadrant B would generate health improvements but there would be a net cost to society or the health services; programmes in Quadrant C would result in additional costs and a deterioration in health status; and, programmes in Quadrant D would generate net benefits but a reduction in health status. For health promotion agencies programmes which were positioned in Quadrant A would receive resources, programmes in Quadrant C should not be resourced while for programmes in Quadrants B and D they would have to resort to other criteria and weights to determine whether these additional costs could be incurred to secure health improvements or whether some health gains could be sacrificed to achieve some monetary return.

Economic evaluation is extremely useful in identifying areas where resources should be allocated, areas which should cease to be funded and areas for which further research needs to be undertaken. However, in the wider context of evaluation of health promotion activities, it must be stressed that economic evaluation is but one of the numerous approaches to be employed and that there are many other criteria, apart from efficiency, against which to judge the worth of such activities.

The impact of economic evaluation on health promotion

The next eight chapters focus on eight areas of health promotion activity in turn. The areas are alcohol, drugs, exercise, mental health, nutrition, safety, sexuality and smoking. Each area is introduced by means of an overview, which provides an insight into the extent of the economic and health problems attributed to the area derived from a variety of literature sources. There follows a detailed review of studies which report the findings of an economic evaluation within the area or which have proposed an economic approach as part of the evaluation process. The lessons which can be gleaned from the literature by health promotion agencies are contained in a summary at the end of each section.

In a number of areas a paucity of appropriate studies was found, due, in the main, to the ongoing debate as to the effectiveness of health promotion in affecting changes in behaviour, in addition to changes in awareness levels. Where, relatively few studies existed, studies which demonstrated potential for economic evaluation or those which had made some passing reference to the need for schemes to be subjected to an economic appraisal as a subsequent phase in the programme's development, were included for review.

Each study is reviewed under a series of headings:

- Problem definition and objectives of investigation.
- Study design and setting.
- Approaches to costing.
- Approaches to outputs and outcomes.
- Conclusions.
- Relevance to health promotion agencies.

In undertaking the literature search the following databases were used:

- Economic literature index.
- Embase.
- Health periodicals database.
- Health planning and administration.
- Medline.

41

- Mental health abstracts.

Search terms used included: health education, health promotion, assessment, evaluation, economic, efficiency, cost, effectiveness, with major descriptors relating to the health promotion areas.

5. Alcohol

Overview

Alcohol has been described as 'our favourite drug' in a report by the Royal College of Psychiatrists (1986) and there is much evidence to support such a claim, with data relating to household expenditure revealing that the amount spent on alcohol is at least equivalent to expenditure on the NHS.

It has been estimated that the social costs associated with alcohol are in the region of £2 billion (Maynard, 1989); while it is difficult to estimate accurately the impact of alcohol on mortality because of poor epidemiological data, the annual alcohol related mortality is between 8,700 and 33,000 and the life years lost are between 185,600 and 224,100 (Godfrey and Maynard, 1992). The impact of alcohol on morbidity is enormous, for example, the impact on inpatient costs range from £88 million to £530 million (Godfrey and Hardman, 1990) while accident and emergency costs have been calculated to be between £18 million and £25 million per year and primary health care costs have been estimated at £2.3 million in 1987 prices (Maynard, 1989). This excludes the high pharmaceutical costs associated with some diseases for which alcohol may be a major contributory factor, for example, hypertension. In addition, up to 20% of all general psychiatric admissions may be alcohol related and alcohol is also linked very closely to a number of other social problems such as crime, domestic violence, child abuse and divorce (Ensor and Godfrey, 1993), injuries (Hingson and Howland, 1993) and a wide range of costs to industry (Powell, 1990).

What is also very evident from the literature are the linkages between the problem areas. Alcohol is closely related with workplace, road traffic, domestic and other forms of accidents and there is a close correlation between alcohol and mental illness, nutritional disorders and so on. It confirms the view that health promotion messages which cross problem boundaries are much more likely to generate efficiencies than those which are highly focused in one particular area.

Review of studies

Reviews of the effectiveness of health promotion activities relating to alcohol problems have provided mixed messages. Moskowitz (1989) states that there was little evidence to suggest that primary prevention programmes were effective although they may become more effective after other policies which alter 'social norms regarding use of beverage alcohol' have been adopted. Grant (1989) suggests that school and other targeted population based campaigns and mass media programmes have not proved effective.

There is evidence however, that some programmes have successfully increased knowledge about alcohol related problems (for example, Rundall and Bruvold, 1988) although whether this translates into changes in consumption is dubious (Rowland and Maynard, 1993). An evaluation of a mass media campaign demonstrated that attitudes towards alcohol use were affected by the campaign but the effects were greater when the campaign was linked to a community programme (Caswell et al., 1990), while Redman et al. (1990) argues that mass media campaigns did not make a major contribution to the combined approach and suggested that the community component, on its own or combined with cheaper methods, would have produced similar behaviour changes.

Powell, M (1990) *Reducing the costs of alcohol in the workplace: the case for employer policies*, **Discussion Paper 68, Centre for Health Economics, University of York.**

Problem definition and objectives of investigation

The paper presented a framework for evaluating the costs and benefits of workplace based interventions in reducing alcohol related problems.

Study design and setting

Cited the cost-effectiveness of many such studies in the USA but argued that the case for increasing the number and type of policies in the UK must be on the basis of cost-efficiency.

44

Approaches to costing

Examined the literature relating to the impact of alcohol on industry and the associated costs and also explained that any policy will result in the firm incurring an increase in current and capital expenditure and therefore unless there were consequential gains in productivity and savings in employment costs then policies would not be practical. Provided an outline of four models (human capital approach, performance monitoring approach, labour market signalling approach and fringe benefits approach) which demonstrated how alcohol policies could be successful in achieving an increase in profitability in the long-term.

Approaches to outputs and outcomes

Highlighted the benefits to employers in terms of improved productivity resulting from such policies but also incorporated other benefits to the employees and society as a whole arising from such schemes.

Conclusions

Strongly argued for careful evaluation of company studies based on the suggested framework and using robust statistical techniques.

Relevance to health promotion agencies

Health promotion agencies could work alongside organisations in designing appropriate work-based strategies and also contribute to the evaluation of such schemes to determine their effectiveness and efficiency.

Tolley, K and Rowland, N (1991) 'Identification of alcohol-related problems in a general hospital setting: a cost-effectiveness evaluation', *British Journal of Addiction***, 86, 429-438.**

Problem definition and objectives of investigation

The study examined the costs of screening patients for alcohol problems.

Study design and setting

The overall aim of the study was to identify the prevalence of patients who drank in excess and to evaluate a screening and health education programme. Data from the study was used for this cost-effectiveness component.

Approaches to costing

The cost-effectiveness component considered the financial consequences of choices between three options for screening patients for alcohol-related problems using junior doctors, nurses or a specialised alcohol worker. The cost of screening was measured as the average time taken to ask a patient a set of questions to discover whether there was evidence of excessive drinking. Cost variations were thus restricted to differentials place don the valuations placed on the time of the three administrators.

Approaches to outputs and outcomes

Six objectives were considered within the cost-effectiveness study. They were lowest cost per screening, greatest numbers screened, greatest rate of positive screening, lowest average cost per positive screening, acceptable marginal cost per additional positive screening, acceptable marginal cost per positive patient admission.

Conclusions

The best option for each of the objectives were: nurses for lowest cost per screening (all patients) and lowest average cost per positive screening (female patients); specialist worker for greatest rate of positive screening (all patients); doctors for lowest average cost per positive screening (male patients and all patients); nurses or specialist worker for greatest number of screenings (all patients), acceptable marginal cost per additional positive screening (female patients) and acceptable marginal cost per positive patient admission (all patients); doctors or specialist worker for acceptable marginal cost per additional positive screening (male patients).

Relevance to health promotion agencies

The study demonstrated that if cost was not an important consideration the specialist alcohol worker was the most effective screening option. This is a function that could be provided by health promotion agencies. However, as soon as cost enters the decision-making arena the situation changes and the article demonstrates that it may be feasible for nurses and doctors to screen patients as part of their 'normal duties', whereas the employment of specialist workers may run the risk of wasted expertise if screening does not fully utilise their work time. Health promotion agencies could lobby for alcohol screening to be included as part of the contract specifications drawn up through purchaser and provider negotiations.

Maynard, A and Godfrey, C (1994) 'Alcohol policy - evaluating the options', *British Medical Bulletin*, 50, 1, 221-230.

Problem definition and objectives of investigation

Considered the range of policy instruments available to reduce the harm from alcohol consumption arguing that, since a reduction could only be achieved at some cost, there was a need for economic appraisals of the options to be undertaken.

Study design and setting

Examined the costs and benefits associated with the options available for reducing alcohol consumption.

Approaches to costing

Argued that the 'production of social cost estimates by economists, while fuelling the political debate, are of little policy relevance when decisions about resource allocation have to be made.'

Approaches to outputs and outcomes

Demonstrated that integrated policies designed to raise taxes in relation to price and income have significant impacts on consumption and if complemented with advertising controls have even larger effects. However, the view was also expressed that the quantity and quality of health care interventions was inadequate.

Conclusions

There is some evidence that minimal interventions which are carefully targeted are cost-effective, but more research is needed, while fiscal and advertising policies have been shown to significantly reduce alcohol if they were implemented. Concluded that 'the industry will lose and oppose change but improvements in health and other aspects of life (e.g. civil order) will be significant'.

Relevance to health promotion agencies

As will be demonstrated with smoking, health promotion activities which are complemented by financial incentives will result in the maximum impact. This study highlights the need for additional work in evaluating the effects of health promotion in reducing alcohol consumption.

Godfrey, C (1994) 'Assessing the cost-effectiveness of alcohol services', *Journal of Mental Health*, 3, 3-21.

Problem definition and objectives of investigation

Discussed the issues involved in undertaking economic evaluations of alcohol interventions and critically reviewed the existing literature.

Study design and setting

Considered the methodology employed in economic appraisal. the question of whether costs of alcohol related treatments may be offset against reductions in medical expenditure and offered suggestions about the most efficient use of resources for the health and social care of those with alcohol related problems.

Approaches to costing

This study was not an economic evaluation but the paper presented a framework for constructing a cost profile which could be utilised as part of an economic evaluation and did consider the issue of whether the costs of alcohol treatment may be offset by health care costs savings.

Approaches to outputs and outcomes

The review of the literature did not produce any clear evidence as to the most efficient approaches.

Conclusions

Very few studies exist which have undertaken a full economic evaluation of alcohol treatments and the author concluded that the 'evidence from both clinical and economic evaluations suggests that, for a majority of problem drinkers, low cost interventions may be as effective as more expensive treatments.'

Relevance to health promotion agencies

On the basis of current evidence it may be necessary that the emphasis is placed on low cost, specifically targeted interventions, while attention is continued to be focused on what constitutes effective measures in this area.

Strategic developments

The literature provides a series of mixed messages with regard to health promotion schemes relating to alcohol consumption. Schemes designed to communicate the 'evils associated with drink' may be successful in increasing knowledge and awareness but the evidence for behaviour change resulting from these approaches is scant, at best. However, there are more positive approaches, for example, the use of work-based settings may prove a useful environment to promote lifestyle change, especially if the costs are borne, in the main, by employers and health promotion agencies is responsible for the design and oversight of the programmes. Further work is needed to compare how psychological interventions can be utilised to minimise the risk associated with excessive alcohol and how social support networks can be used to prevent relapse. Hospitals have been shown to be effective as screening settings for detecting excessive consumption and, it may be of some benefit for health promotion agencies to liaise with provider units to establish programmes which were administered as part of the normal procedures within hospital at entry and exit.

There is a strong lobby for linking the health promotion messages with a fiscal approach so as to attach a financial incentive to the health campaign, while for health promotion agencies the lesson may be that low-cost programmes are the most efficient at this time, especially when part of a wider lifestyle approach.

6. Drugs

Overview

'The use of illicit drugs like the use of legal addictive substances such as alcohol and tobacco, imposes uncompensated costs on society' (Maynard et al., 1987). Griffin (1992) suggested that by 1992 it was widely acknowledged that there were more than 150,000 regular opiate users in the UK. The total costs to society resulting from drug abuse are difficult to estimate with any degree of precision because of the dearth of any reliable epidemiological data. However, the extent of the problem is not confined to the UK and the developed world but represents a major international problem which affects almost every country in the world.

The many health problems and deaths associated with drug abuse are the result of complex interactions between the drugs (and their pharmaceutical and toxicological properties), the users (and their personalities and health state) and the settings in which the drugs are taken. However, while the illicit drug market has resulted in fortunes being made for drug barons on the one hand, and enormous social problems to individuals, families and communities alike on the other, it is virtually impossible to estimate the costs of drug use on society (Sutton and Maynard, 1992). These authors repeat earlier claims that a regular national survey of drug use would be a useful source of additional information and conclude that 'without such data the agencies of government will continue to assert that the drug problem is 'considerable' and their efforts to contain it are 'successful' and there will be inadequate evidence to substantiate such claims. At present government is spending hundreds of millions of pounds on a policy problem whose magnitude and trends are unknown. It should not be surprised that its success appears to be limited but taxpayers should be concerned that their money is spent with so little regard to 'value of money issues.'

Review of studies

While there are some studies which have examined the efficiency of supply side policy measures (for example, Wagstaff and Maynard, 1988; Sutton and Maynard, 1994) there is a paucity of investigations which have considered the efficiency of demand side measures. This can be attributed to the serious lack of effectiveness data which exists. There is an abundance of studies which have explored the effectiveness of educational programmes on drug abuse (for example, Bagert-Drowns, 1988; Green and Kelley, 1989; Bruvold, 1990; Coggans et al., 1991; Becker et al., 1992; Ellickson et al., 1993; Ennett et al., 1994) and they all report that the effects of the programmes are relatively small, or have some impact on knowledge and attitudes but are unsuccessful in changing behaviour. Programmes which seek to focus on social influence may be more successful in reducing the motivation to begin using drugs (Donaldson et al., 1994).

The result is that virtually no economic evaluations of health promotion activities relating to drug abuse were produced by the literature search and the studies used in this review therefore demonstrate how economic evaluations may be utilised in this area rather than examples of where they have been used.

Orlandi, M A et al. (1990) 'Computer-assisted strategies for substance abuse prevention: opportunities and barriers', *Journal of Consulting and Clinical Psychology,* **58, 4, 425-31.**

Problem definition and objectives of investigation

Presented an analysis of the potential role of computer-assisted strategies in preventing substance abuse.

Study design and setting

Considered the role of substance use prevention within the context of adolescent development, the opportunities afforded by computer technology, the barriers which might inhibit its utilisation and the need for adequate evaluation of the strategy.

Approaches to costing

No explicit reference made to costs but implicit within the discussion was the notion that computers were becomingly increasingly involved in many aspects of today's society, including primary and secondary school education systems. It is contended that computer approaches can be more readily be adapted to meet the needs of individual students. The issue of cost constraint was raised but it was argued that barriers related to cost 'will become less relevant' over time.

Approaches to outputs and outcomes

Offered suggested benefits which would merge from use of a computer based prevention strategy.

Conclusions

The authors, arguing from the standpoint that 'substance abuse will continue to present a formidable challenge to the health and well-being of our nation,' stressed the need for effective prevention initiatives. In this light they argued that inter-disciplinary approaches were desired between those organisations involved in the research, development and communication of programmes and with those agencies who were involved with the recipient of such programmes, if 'intervention strategies are the be efficiently derived.'

Relevance to health promotion agencies

Opportunities may exist for health promotion agencies to work alongside the 'communication agencies' in the development of relevant software packages which can be both effective and efficient methods of communicating the perils of substance use to school-children.

Sarvela, P D and Ford, T D (1993) 'An evaluation of a substance abuse education program for Mississippi Delta pregnant adolescents', *Journal of School Health*, 63, 3, 147-152.

Problem definition and objectives of investigation

The study examined the effects of a substance abuse education programme on knowledge, attitudes and behaviour and the consequential impact on new-borns.

Study design and setting

A non-equivalent control group was used as the study design and subjects assigned to the groups on the basis of area of residence.

Approaches to costing

The education programme was incorporated within the prenatal programmes for the subjects and the only costs incurred were the materials used in the programme.

Approaches to outputs and outcomes

The findings demonstrated an increase in knowledge between the pre-test and post-test surveys with some evidence of greater decrease in drug use amongst the experimental group.

Conclusions

The study itself recommended the use of cost-effectiveness and cost-benefit studies to encompass a broader evaluation of what appeared to be an effective strategy of prenatal substance abuse education.

Relevance to health promotion agencies

This study indicates that targeting of particular groups can be beneficial in securing effectiveness. The linking of educational programmes to other interventions can also reduce the costs involved and thereby secure a cost-effective approach.

Plotnick, R D (1994) 'Applying benefit-cost analysis to substance use prevention programs', *International Journal of the Addictions,* **29, 3, 339-359.**

Problem definition and objectives of investigation

Argued strongly for the use of cost-effectiveness and cost-benefit analysis in the evaluation of substance use prevention programmes.

Study design and setting

Presented a case for the use of the economic techniques and demonstrated how this could be accomplished within the area of substance use prevention. Reference was also made to a scheme designed to prevent relapse into drug use by a group of methadone treatment parents and lower the risk that the children will become substance users.

Approaches to costing

Discussed direct and indirect costs associated with such programmes in terms of opportunity costs and stressed the need for identification, at least, of all costs.

Approaches to outputs and outcomes

Distinguished between monetary and non-monetary benefits emerging from such programmes and suggested that findings should be tested against a range of discount rates.

Conclusions

Argued for consideration to be given to the equity aspects resulting from such programmes and emphasised that 'even if funds are not sufficient to conduct a careful benefit-cost analysis, the organising concepts can help administrators and evaluators think more systematically about a program's activities and impacts.'

Relevance to health promotion agencies

This study confirms the recognition by health promotion agencies that programmes should be subjected to rigorous evaluation which includes notions of efficiency amongst its criteria.

Strategic developments

There appears to be very limited evidence to base any firm judgements upon in this area, but there it would appear that a collaborative approach across relevant agencies should be adopted in this area, so as to minimise costs and avoiding duplication of effort, with the targeting of high risk groups for intervention proving to be the most efficient use of resources.

7. Exercise

Overview

There is considerable literature associating the health benefits to be derived from exercise. Compared with a sedentary lifestyle, regular participation in exercise improves body functioning, for example, circulation, strength, stamina and joint mobility. There is convincing evidence of the preventive effect of exercise on the risk factors associated with coronary heart disease, cerebrovascular diseases, osteoporosis and hip fracture, diabetes mellitus and mental illness and it is also effective in moderating the effects of other health damaging behaviour, such as smoking and poor diet. In addition, there may be other indirect benefits as a result of exercise. For example, Block et al. (1987) found that, although exercise had not yet been shown to prevent fractures, improved muscle tone would almost certainly reduce the likelihood of falling, particularly amongst the elderly. It should also be remembered that exercise is potentially a two-edged sword, with an increased risk of injury and accidents occurring as a result of increased participation in exercise and sporting activities. What remains unclear is the amount and type of exercise required to achieve benefit (Elwood et al., 1993; Ebrahim and Williams, 1992), although in the USA one study has sought to prescribe a exercise programme which maximises the benefits and minimises the risks attached to an exercise and regular physical activity (Levine and Balady, 1993).

However, it has been estimated that 74% of men and 68% of women are below the age adjusted activity levels required to achieve all the health benefits of exercise (Allied Dunbar, 1992) and therefore it is an area where health promotion agencies need to be involved.

Review of studies

While a number of studies emerged which demonstrated the contribution of exercise to generating improvements in health and reducing risks associated with a range of diseases, there were very few studies which considered the efficiency of interventions designed to promote the benefits of increased exercise amongst the population.

Four major studies emerged as suitable for analysis. Three are the results of investigations undertaken in USA, while one is a review of the literature which examined the value of promoting health through exercise.

Nicholl, J P, Coleman, P and Brazier, J E (1994) 'Health and health care costs and benefits of exercise', *PharmacoEconomics*, 5, 2, 109-122.

Problem definition and objectives of investigation

The study aimed to assess the value of promoting health through exercise.

Study design and setting

Literature searches were undertaken to derive the estimates of relative risk of those who exercised regularly compared with those who did not. This was done for a variety of diseases where there was sound evidence of the benefits of exercise, in order to estimate the healthcare costs which could be prevented if the whole population exercised.

Approaches to costing

A cost-of-illness approach adopted with the cost of each admission estimated as the product of the average length of stay for the disease category and an average cost per day for an admission to a UK NHS hospital.

Approaches to outputs and outcomes

Estimates of the exercise-related reduction in the risk of each disease, and hence reductions in mortality and morbidity and potential savings in treatment costs, were considered against the estimated risks and costs of exercise-related illness, injury and death.

Conclusions

Medical costs as a result of younger adults (ages 15-44) taking part in sport and exercise exceed the costs that would be saved by disease-preventing effects of that exercise. In older adults, on the other hand, the estimated cost saved in disease prevention by taking part in exercise greatly outweighed the costs incurred through sports injury.

Relevance to health promotion agencies

It is acknowledged that many of the estimates used in the study are crude and that the negative benefits for the younger age group are due in the main to the relatively high risk sports and exercise that they engage in. The authors acknowledged that 'on the information available, it seems that the principal benefit from exercising at younger ages lies in the development of exercise behaviour patterns that will remain in later life.' The message for health promotion agencies is that while exercise for the over 45 age group would appear to be cost-effective, there is a need to promote low-risk exercise patterns for those in the younger age bracket. However, even in a segment of the older group, there is on-going debate as to how much exercise is necessary, for how long and of what type. An evaluation of the Health Education Authority Look After Yourself exercise package amongst two groups of people (aged 58-89), reached the conclusion that such questions remain unanswered and that the effects of mild to moderate exercise need further systematic research in larger, controlled studies (Ebrahim and Williams, 1992).

Kaplan, R M, Atkins, C J and Wilson, D K (1988) 'The cost-utility of diet and exercise interventions in non-insulin-dependent diabetes mellitus', *Health Promotion*, 2, 4, 331-340.

Problem definition and objectives of investigation

The study sought to evaluate the cost-utility of behavioural interventions for non-insulin dependent diabetes mellitus (NIDDM) patients over a short-term period of 18 months.

Study design and setting

A series of public announcements, newspaper notices and referrals from physicians resulted in 87 people attending orientation meetings at which they were offered opportunity to participate in an experimental study considering the effect of weight loss on the control of NIDDM. Seventy-six subjects met all necessary diagnostic criteria and were randomly assigned to one of four groups, one to receive a dietary intervention, one to receive an exercise programme, one to receive the dietary programme and the exercise programme and one to receive a series of ten lectures focusing on diabetic care.

The outcome comparisons between the four groups did not form part of this article, having been commented upon in previous studies, but the authors explained that the cost-utility analysis would be undertaken on the most effective intervention, that of the combined diet and exercise programme in comparison to the education programme, as the control.

Approaches to costing

Only direct costs to the organisations involved were included in the study and indirect costs, in terms of patient time and resources and side effects associated with the diet and exercise programme were not included. Average clinical charges based on 1986 rates were used rather than the more reliable data generated if the costs had been based on actual resources used by the patients undertaking the programme(s).

Approaches to outputs and outcomes

The study used the Quality of Well-being Scale to compare the outcomes generated by the diet and exercise intervention in comparison to the education programme over an eighteen month period, gathering data at initial interview, 3 months, 6 months, 12 months and 18 months.

Conclusions

The investigation revealed that the diet and exercise programme yielded an additional 0.092 well-years over the education programme which when related to the average cost of $1,000 produced a result of $10,870 per additional well year (1986 prices). A sensitivity analysis was undertaken to test the findings against a number of assumptions. If the intervention had been half as effective as observed the cost-utility would be $21,740 while if discount rates of 5% and 10% had been utilised to counter the effect of time the estimates would have been $11,690 and $12,500 respectively. The argument that discount rates were not needed because of the limited time scale considered by the investigation are borne out by the sensitivity analysis.

The authors concluded that 'investments in behavioural interventions produce benefits at a cost quite comparable to many widely advocated health care alternatives. We encourage the use of cost-utility analysis for the evaluation of other behavioural and biomedical interventions in health care.'

Relevance to health promotion agencies

The study demonstrates the attractiveness of combining nutritional and exercise strategies in this particular setting, at least, but it does suggest that a labour intensive behavioural intervention can generate significant health gain at relatively low cost. however, the study was relatively small scale and had a clearly defined target group, features which may be more difficult for health promotion agencies to work within.

Hatziandreu, E I et al. (1988) 'A cost-effectiveness analysis of exercise as a health promotion activity', *American Journal of Public Health*, 78, 11, 1417-1421.

Problem definition and objectives of investigation

The study arose out of what the authors claimed was the convincing empirical support for the cardiovascular benefits of exercise which had led the medical profession to recognise and prescribe exercise as a preventive and rehabilitative activity.

The objective was to use cost-effectiveness analysis to estimate the health and economic implications of exercise in preventing coronary heart disease (CHD).

Study design and setting

Two hypothetical cohorts of 1,000 men (one with exercise and one without) were followed for 30 years to observe differences in the number of CHD events, life expectancy and quality-adjusted life expectancy. The impact of exercise was based on age-specific incidence rates drawn from the Framingham Heart Study.

Approaches to costing

The study employed a relatively thorough approach to costing by including the direct costs of exercise (purchase of equipment and counselling costs), the indirect costs of exercise (time foregone, which was accorded different valuations based on the extent to which participants enjoy exercise), the direct medical costs of injury (physician time and X-rays), the indirect cost of injury based on the average hours of work lost because of injury, direct costs to the health services associated with CHD and earnings lost due to disability and premature death (indirect costs of CHD).

Approaches to outputs and outcomes

Health outcomes, CHD cases/deaths averted and life years gained were predicted using life expectancy tables and epidemiological data on the relationship between exercise and CHD incidence.

Conclusions

The findings generated were that the cost/QALY gained was $11,313; the cost/Year of Life gained was $27,851; the cost/CHD case averted was $76,760 and the cost/CHD death averted was $250,836. The authors also concluded that there was a differential of $6 million in total costs for the cohort of exercisers over the non-exercising cohort. Extensive testing of the results were carried out and the authors also commented that if exercise was only undertaken if there was some enjoyment from it or at least people were indifferent to it, then the total costs would fall to $23 million, a net benefit of $2.7 million. The authors conclude that 'exercise is a cost-effective way of lowering the risk of CHD' for those who enjoy the pleasure and benefits of exercise but accept that the findings are based on a number of assumptions and the 'best available data.'

Relevance to health promotion agencies

The study suffers from the lack of firm evidence of the link between exercise and health benefits. However, for those who enjoy participation in exercise there is evidence that it may be a cost-effective means of generating health gains, although this may have to be balanced against the findings of Nicholl et al. (1994). The same cannot be said of those who are non-exercisers and the problem for health promotion agencies, and others, is that such people may display other 'potential lifestyle problems.' For such people specific health promotion activities may not have the desired impact unless accompanied by some financial incentives to alter their behaviour patterns. For example, it has been shown that taxation policies can, with smoking cessation programmes, increase the impact on smoking prevalence (Townsend, 1994). It may therefore be attractive for health promotion agencies to liaise with other relevant organisations to try and establish a system of financial inducements to engage in some form of exercise, by linking a smoking cessation competition to 'free' access to local leisure facilities, or offering taxation incentives to those organisations who provide fitness related programmes for their employees, or enabling free access to leisure complexes for the unemployed, etc.

Shephard, R J (1992) 'A critical analysis of work-site fitness programs and their postulated economic benefits', *Medicine and Science in Sports and Exercise,* **24, 3, 354-370.**

Problem definition and objectives of investigation

The study examined the content of work-site fitness programmes, their postulated benefits, factors modifying the effectiveness of the programmes, the costs associated with the programmes and the relationship between costs and the effectiveness of the programmes.

Study design and setting

A literature review of work-site fitness and lifestyle programmes in North America to assess their impact in terms of employee turnover, productivity, absenteeism, medical costs, etc.

Approaches to costing

While it is recognised that a full economic evaluation must consider such issues as opportunity costs to participants and marginal costs the concentration is on the costs to the organisation, in terms of promotion, facilities, equipment and professional leadership, which in total varied between $200 to $2,000 per participant.

Approaches to outputs and outcomes

The study commented on the susceptibility, participation rate, response rate and continued employment by the organisation as indicators of the extent of effectiveness of programmes in seeking to accomplish the benefits highlighted above.

Conclusions

Tentatively concluded that activities that can be built into the normal day of the employee (for example, walking or cycling to and from work) may prove more acceptable and more cost-effective than formal work-site classes.

Relevance to health promotion agencies

There appears to be some doubt as to whether workplace interventions are cost-effective but it has to be remembered that the review was of North American situations. The method of funding health care in the UK is very different from that in the USA and although there is increasing evidence of employers taking a more proactive role in the health of their employees through private health care schemes, there is also a role for health promotion agencies to continue to impress upon employers the need for a fit and healthy workforce. The study also highlights the substantial benefits that can be acquired relative to the costs incurred in how the working day is organised and how travel to and from work is organised. Health promotion agencies can continue to emphasise the benefits from such exercise.

Strategic developments

The literature review highlights the debate surrounding the use of exercise as an efficient means of generating health gain. The promotion of exercise at a young age is probably an efficient strategy in that it can prove habit forming and be beneficial at a later stage of life. Exercise programmes need to be carefully constructed because of the risk factors involved while the integration of exercise as part of broader programmes may prove to be more beneficial. especially for those who get no consumption benefits, such as enjoyment, from participating in such activities.

There is also evidence to suggest that for health promotion agencies, liaison with other agencies, who might bear substantial elements of the costs involved, would be an efficient strategy to employ in seeking to communicate the benefits of participating in and the health benefits produced by low-risk exercise programmes.

8. Mental health

Overview

The available evidence indicates that much mental illness is undiagnosed and untreated (Eisenberg, 1992; West, 1992), which makes any estimate of the costs of the disorder incomplete and problematic. West (1992), for example, estimates that the total cost of depression to the NHS was £333m; that UK family doctors diagnose two million cases of depression each year; that as many as 1 in 8 patients seen by general practitioners suffer from depressive symptoms, with a similar number either missed or misdiagnosed. The Mental Health Foundation state that expenditure on treatment and care for the mentally ill represents around 8% of total NHS revenue spending and amounts to over £2,000 million (1989 prices). They also claim that mental health is as common as heart disorders, three times as common as cancer, over 3,000 times more common than AIDS, that it kills four times as many people as are killed on our roads and that it represents 17% (that is 71 million) of the working days lost due to sickness (Thompson and Pudney, 1990).

Review of studies

One of the major emergents from the literature search in this area was the extent of inter-relationship between mental health problems and the extent of participation in 'health damaging' activities. This study is not the venue to discuss the extent of these causal relationships or whether such lifestyle patterns are reflective of a range of complex social, economic and environmental factors. Nevertheless, it is worth commencing this section with reference to a conference paper, which does not meet the criteria of economic evaluation and is not discussed within the framework adopted for other studies, but poses some highly important issues in seeking to assess the economic effectiveness of health promotion in the field of mental health.

Albee, G (1994) 'The fourth revolution' in Trent, D R and Reed, C *Promotion of mental health: Volume 3-1993*, **Avebury: Aldershot.**

The title of Albee's paper stemmed from his belief that the fourth mental health revolution would involve a major shift towards efforts at prevention. He recounted that the Commission on the Prevention of Mental/Emotional Disorders of the Mental Health Association (1986) took testimony from a wide range of experts from various fields in order to produce a monograph that would stimulate programming to eventually reduce the incidence of mental and emotional disabilities. During one of the sessions the following question was asked by one of the members:

> If we had just one prevention programme we could put into place, and knew it would succeed, which one would that be?

After some hours of discussion the answer was provided:

> We would choose a programme that would ensure that every baby born would be a healthy, full-term infant who was welcomed into the world by parent(s) who were financially secure, who had decided in advance that they (she) wanted the child, and who had planned for her or his conception and birth...If every child arrived under these conditions the rate of mental and emotional problems in the next generation would be reduced significantly.

He also referred to the footnotes added by members of the Commission. Selecting those of major relevance to this study produced :

> It would be wonderful if the mother were breast fed by an adequately nourished mother.

> The mother (and father) should not be a smoker, a heavy user of alcohol or other drugs before or during pregnancy and subsequent to the arrival of the child.

The mother would have an adequate pre-natal health care including a diet adequate in protein, calcium, iron and other essential nutrients.

Other comments included issues relating to social, economic and educational factors. In concluding, he presented a model for reducing the incidence of psychopathology, which amounts to reducing one of the more noxious agents (defined as organic factors, stress factors and exploitation) expressed as the numerator of the formula and increasing one or more of the sources of host resistance in the denominator (defined as social and coping skills, self-esteem enhancement and support systems).

He presented a powerful argument for preventive schemes in mental health stating that there is an '...accumulating body of evidence that prevention programmes actually reduce the incidence of children's mental disorders...' whereas '...even effective treatment doesn't reduce incidence... the only way to reduce significantly the incidence of mental and emotional disorders is through primary prevention.'

This view was also expressed by Barker et al. (1993), who, in an evaluation of a television series aimed at preventing mental illness, claimed that 'preventive services frequently have the additional advantage of employing a cost effective one-to-many approach rather than the one-to-one approach of traditional clinical work.'

However, the powerful case advocated by Albee (1994) also pose potentially sensitive issues for the strategic direction of health promotion agencies. He highlighted, for example, the impact of unemployment on mental health, resulting in increased rates of child and wife abuse, increased consumption of alcohol, depression and social withdrawal and argues that 'prevention strategies must involve intervention at the level of social variables.'

The search of literature did not reveal many studies which examined the issues from an economic perspective and therefore some of the studies discussed below should be viewed in a slightly different light. The studies reviewed are taken from different settings, the workplace, primary health care, specialist services and direct contacts with the public.

Burton, W N (1991) 'Value-managed mental health benefits', *Journal of Occupational Medicine*, 33, 3, 311-313.

Problem definition and objectives of investigation

In order to counter the escalating mental health care usage and costs by its staff the First National Bank of Chicago introduced, in 1984, an Employee Assistance Program designed to provide quality and cost-effective mental health care services for employees and their dependents, through prevention, early intervention and appropriate care of mental health problems.

Study design and setting

The study examined the impact of the programme on the costs to the organisation's medical plan, compared impatient psychiatric utilisation and costs and days lost through short-term psychiatric disability.

Approaches to costing

Nothing was reported of the costs of establishing the programme nor of indirect costs to employees.

Approaches to outputs and outcomes

It was shown that mental health costs fell from 14% of the total medical plan costs in 1984 to 12% in 1988, inpatient mental health costs (not adjusted for inflation) fell from $953,596 in 1984 to $390,791 in 1988 during a time when overall health care costs were increasing by some 10% per year and there was a reduction in the average length of psychiatric short-term disability episodes for employees.

Conclusions

It is claimed that primary prevention and early intervention, together with benefit plan management results in an effective response to the rising demand and cost of mental health care.

Relevance to health promotion agencies

While the above findings are impressive, there is also evidence to suggest that they should be treated with some degree of caution. Warner et al. (1988), in a review of the literature of workplace health promotion programmes, found that the research base for the cost-benefit and cost-effectiveness of employee assistance programs was extremely limited (although they concentrated in the main on alcohol and drug abuse) and there was no research base for stress management issues in the workplace.

What is noteworthy for health promotion agencies, however, is that where a large proportion of the costs can be incurred by other agencies (such as industry and commerce) it does enable the limited resources of health promotion agencies to be channelled into areas and activities where most benefit can be derived. Liaison with employers is part of the case developed by Jenkins (1993), who listed some of the occupational consequences of psychological illness as sickness absence, impaired relations with colleagues, reduced work performance, accidents and labour turnover. He argued that 'all of these have measurable social and economic costs' and can be used in the decision as to whether it is cost effective to initiate preventive strategies in the workplace. He proposed that such policies could be instigated at primary (preventing illness from happening in the first place), secondary (early detection and prompt management of depressions and anxiety) and tertiary (rehabilitation back to work of those who have had a fairly severe illness) stages.

Health promotion agencies may wish to consider taking on a proactive role in developing relationships with employers and other agencies to establish policies at each stage.

Scott, A I F and Freeman, C P L (1992) 'Edinburgh primary care depression study: treatment outcome, patient satisfaction and cost after 16 weeks', *British Medical Journal*, 304, 883-887.

Problem definition and objectives of investigation

This study aimed to compare the clinical efficacy, patient satisfaction and cost of three specialist treatments for depressive illness with routine care by GPs in primary care.

Study design and setting

One hundred and twenty one patients, aged between 18 and 65 years suffering depressive illness were prospectively, randomly allocated to amitriptyline prescribed by a psychiatrist, cognitive behaviour therapy from a clinical psychologist, counselling and case work by a social worker or routine care by a GP.

Approaches to costing

Costing was confined to face to face contacts with professionals and drug costs.

Approaches to outputs and outcomes

Depression amongst patients was assessed using the Hamilton rating scale by raters at week 0, week 4 and week 16 and recovery rates were calculated at 4 and 16 weeks. Patients were also asked to evaluate their treatment and compliance with their prescribed drug dose.

Conclusions

While marked improvements in depressive symptoms occurred in all treatment groups over 16 weeks and psychological treatments, especially social work counselling were most positively evaluated, the additional costs associated with specialist treatments of new episodes were not commensurate with their clinical superiority over routine GP care.

Relevance to health promotion agencies

Sheldon et al. (1993) confirmed the view that larger scale evaluation is required to guide resource allocation decisions relating to social work and counselling interventions by health visitors in primary care setting, while they also expressed the view that the evidence for the effectiveness of counsellors being employed in general practice was ambiguous.

With regard to strategies designed to reduce suicide it is not possible to accurately predict which depressed patients will attempt to commit suicide (Freemantle et al., 1993) and, according to Sheldon et al. (1993), strategies designed to reduce suicide 'must be aimed at all those diagnosed with major depression, and cannot be aimed at a subset potentially at high risk.'

Rutz, W et al. (1992) 'Cost-benefit analysis of an educational program for general practitioners by the Swedish Committee for the Prevention and Treatment of Depression', *Acta Psychiatrica Scandinavia,* **85, 457-464.**

Problem definition and objectives of investigation

The study described a cost-benefit analysis of an educational programme on the diagnosis and treatment of depressive orders for all general practitioners in Gotland.

Study design and setting

All general practitioners were invited to participate in 2 two-day educational programmes in 1983 and 1984 and approximately 90% of all permanently employed practitioners took part in the training.

Approaches to costing

Costs of the intervention, including preparation and execution of the programme, plus the costs of time of the teachers and doctors, were quantified and added to the increased drug costs. It was assumed that there would be no changes to the primary care routines and medical costs resulting from the programme.

Approaches to outputs and outcomes

A range of benefits were considered in the study. It was assumed that there would be a reduction in in-patient care, a reduction in sickness and absence from work and benefits from a reduction in the number of suicides.

Conclusions

Total costs for the programme were estimated to be around SEK370,000. This did not include changes in drug costs (there was an increase in the number of antidepressants but major reductions in the number of tranquilisers and sedatives) which meant a saving in drug costs of SEK227,000 plus in-patient care savings of SEK 11,250,000. Indirect benefits were estimated to be in the order of SEK144,000,000 which produced a net overall benefit of SEK155,500,000.

A sensitivity analysis was undertaken and if the most conservative estimates were used the net benefit still amounted to SEK17,300,000.

Relevance to health promotion agencies

This has obvious implications for health promotion agencies. Working alongside primary care workers in order to develop policies and activities aimed at minimising the extent of depression within society would appear to be the way forward. The nature of the programme should be carefully considered because it has been shown that, one possible approach, routine screening for depression may not be suitable because of a lack of conclusive evidence that treatment improved outcome and also because evaluation of suicide risk by primary care givers has not been evaluated (Canadian Task Force on the Periodic Health Examination, 1990).

Light, D and Bailey, V (1993) 'Pound foolish', *Health Service Journal.* 11 February, 16-18.

Problem definition and objectives of investigation

This reported the ways in which educational gain, employment gain, law-and-order gain, welfare gain as well as health gain were generated by investment in mental health services for disturbed and abused children.

Study design and setting

The findings from a single case study were translated into a purchasing plan based on epidemiological and demographic data and linked to budgetary information in North West Thames Health Authority.

Approaches to costing

The study examined a series of costed diagnostically related service packages for child mental health services, while recognising the probability of underestimation given that costs are also borne by other agencies and families.

Approaches to outputs and outcomes

Savings produced by early intervention and treatment in financial terms, health gain, prevention of poverty, crimes, injuries and self-induced illnesses were assessed.

Conclusions

It is worth quoting directly from the article. 'This case vignette comes from the first needs-based purchasing plan for child mental health services for Britain. It is one of the most difficult cases, and cost several thousand pounds to treat. In return, a second generation of beating, reliance on benefits and crime was stopped, and a third generation was saved from perpetuating this family syndrome. The immediate and direct costs of social service, probation and the children's home (about £72,000 a year for the two children) ended. Medical costs, present and projected, are down substantially. Charles' father now pays taxes on a reasonably paid job. Besides health gain and the prevention of poverty, crimes, injuries and self-induced illnesses, a 10-fold return in investment was made short term, and probably 100-fold long term.'

Relevance to health promotion agencies

The major lesson to be gleaned from this study is the need to examine both sides of the efficiency coin and not just the one side of costs - hence the title of the article. However, it also points to the need for close collaboration between all agencies and this is perhaps where health promotion agencies can act as a focal point for agencies involved in the purchasing and provision of services for children, and people in general. suffering from or likely to be affected by mental illness. Obviously, seeking to prevent mental illness in the first place is of high priority, but there is also a need to instigate secondary and tertiary preventive schemes to restrict and contain the potentially damaging consequences of mental illness if it is allowed to proceed through its normal course.

Hobson, S and Cameron, I (1994) 'Feeling good in Burley: Evaluation of a week to promote mental health' in Trent, D R and Reed, C *Promotion of mental health: Volume 3-1993*, **Avebury: Aldershot.**

Problem definition and objectives of investigation

In many senses it is rather unfair to include this particular study as it did not include in its study objectives any consideration of the economics of the project. However, comments on it will serve to illustrate how beneficial such an analysis would have been.

The objectives of the project focused on:

- increasing the public's awareness of their own mental health;
- giving some introduction to coping skills which might be expected to support this;
- developing inter-agency networks to make individuals more of the aware of the work of others;
- development of skills in mental health promotion at a local level, and
- ensuring that mental health promotion gained appropriate recognition in the work of local agencies.

This last objective cries out for an economic component to be included in the evaluation framework given pressure on resources and the need to establish priorities.

Study design and setting

The study was an evaluation of a pilot project in a small area of Leeds designed to raise the profile of mental health promotion on the agendas of the various agencies involved, to stimulate inter-agency work in the field and to pilot a variety of methods of approaching the general public.

The evaluation was undertaken on the basis of records kept from the start of the project and sought to explore the process of its development, the final programme presented, the impact of the programme and outcomes.

Approaches to costing

The only reference to costs was the funding of £5,000 obtained from Leeds Health Authority, with no attempt made to quantify and measure the direct costs of establishing and implementing the programme, yet alone the indirect costs associated with the programme - identified as tensions between agencies, lack of role definitions and responsibilities. etc.

Approaches to outputs and outcomes

The impact of the programme were identified in terms of attendance rates, opinions of organisers and participants acquired via short, self-administered questionnaires and the extent of media coverage and how the messages correlated with those intended.

Outcomes were listed, although not quantified, and included mental health promotion being funded through joint finance in the district; the legitimisation of mental health promotion within the district health promotion unit and a named person being given responsibility; development of a mental health promotion strategy; construction of a resource pack, which draws on the experiences gained. In addition, the lessons learned from the initiative were documented and highlighted for further consideration.

Conclusions

The evaluation concluded that the campaign 'was felt to be successful' and that the 'involvement of local people and workers in the planning and implementation of the week...was felt to have improved the quality, impact and the scope of the week's events.'

The dearth of relevant studies in the field of mental health promotion has meant that this type of study has received more attention than probably warranted. However, there are lessons to be gleaned from it for health promotion agencies. In the first place, it provides further evidence for the targeting of campaigns (Albee, 1990) - the chosen area of Burley had been identified from a 1990 health needs assessment as one with high levels of stress and depression amongst its residents, especially young mothers, carers and ethnic minorities. Secondly, it emphasises the need for clear aims and objectives at all stages of a campaign so that the tensions between agencies, which might have diluted the impact of the programme, were avoided. However, it must be remembered that the lack of attention to costings and the nature of the outcomes listed do not enable any examination of the relative efficiency of such an approach.

Woodward, R (1993) 'Evaluating the Wirral Health Mind project: Looking at information uptake and participants' resposes', in Trent, D R and Reed, C *Promotion of mental health: Volume 2-1992*, Avebury: Aldershot.

Problem definition and objectives of investigation

Wirral Health Mind week was a project designed to educate the public about mental health and maximise the coping skills of the community. It had been planned for twelve months and took place in September 1991 in a large shopping precinct in Birkenhead.

Study design and setting

The evaluation consisted of two parts. The first was an observational study of the days to record the total number and type of leaflets taken by the public, the contact with the displays by members of the public and engagement or enquiries on mental health issues by member of the public. The second part took the form of a retrospective study to the people involved in the project to assess the level of practical involvement, satisfaction with the involvement, attitudes towards mental health and the effect on likely future interaction.

Approaches to costing

The costs of the project were based on estimates of average time spent by the various personnel on the project. The estimated figure was £23,000 which was based on 233 working days. No costs were included for costs of materials, displays, etc.

Approaches to outputs and outcomes

Output and outcome measures were restricted to the number of leaflets (nearly 13,000 on different topics), contacts with the public (3,392), of whom 2,078 made enquiries or engaged volunteers staffing the stands and levels of satisfaction with involvement and contact by the personnel involved.

Conclusions

The opening statement indicates that the 'Wirral Healthy Mind Week was a very successful multi-agency initiative which promoted interaction with the local community on mental health issues.' However, the conclusion also points to the need to introduce specifically focused initiatives for young people, men and ethnic minorities, who were more reluctant to engage in the approach adopted in order to enhance the broad spectrum of a general mental health week.

Relevance to health promotion agencies

Again the lack of an economics angle was problematic but health promotion agencies should be aware that inter-agency collaboration requires much investment if its is to be successful. The study reported that 'paid workers from medium-sized organisations gave most time and felt most involved and satisfied. Members of larger organisations, although equally involved, reported less satisfaction. Perhaps, interestingly, users of services and voluntary groups seemed very committed in terms of response rate, but also reported slightly more cautious results. They felt able to contribute less time, felt less satisfied and less optimistic about the true success of the project.'

Strategic developments

Within this area, it would appear that the role for health promotion agencies is to act as a focal point for relevant agencies, in seeking to prevent the on-set of mental illness and to deal speedily with the illness on diagnosis. The difficulty, however, in developing a strategy is that many of the causal factors are social and the prevention of mental illness requires a strategy that combines economic, political. social and health promotion measures. There have been contributions to the literature which highlight effective intervention in mental health promotion and how to develop successful interventions (Hodgson et al., 1996; Hosman and Veltman, 1994) but very little on the economic impact of such initiatives.

As with the other areas of health promotion considered, there is some evidence that liaison working with and developing educational programmes for primary health care teams would be an efficient use of resources, as would the use of workplaces for the implementation of programmes designed to minimise the on-set of debilitating mental problems.

9. Nutrition

Overview

Nutritional disorders, such as obesity, anorexia nervosa and bulimia nervosa have significant implications on mortality are associated with considerable morbidity and mortality. 'On a planet where millions die of starvation or the complications of malnutrition each year, it is a tragic paradox that in some of the world's great agricultural heartlands...individuals are damaging and even killing themselves by eating too much, or too little, or alternating between these unhealthy behaviours in a pathological way' (West, 1987).

The cost of such nutritional disorders are extremely difficult to predict, and as with most of the other areas being investigated in the report, any such cost estimates only form a narrow tip of what are potentially large icebergs. For example, one estimate of the cost to the NHS of anorexia nervosa was over £4 million per annum (West, 1994a) but this did not include costs involved in providing psychotherapy, group, family, behavioural and cognitive therapy, the increased risk of suicide and treating those who were unsuccessful in their attempts, the effects of lost production due to inability to work and the economic significance of the loss of a young life.

The total economic cost of obesity in USA has been estimated to be $69 million in 1990 (Wolf and Colditz, 1994) while the cost to the NHS of obesity has been estimated to be in excess of £165 million (West, 1994b). These estimates are based on the immense costs of diseases in which obesity is a risk factor. Other private costs in the form of slimming and diet products purchased by those who perceive themselves to be overweight should also be taken into account. Studies have shown that being overweight during adolescence also has social and psychological consequences, including an effect on school performance, college acceptance and psychological functioning, while overweight young adults are less likely to get married and have lower household incomes in their early adult life than their non-overweight counterparts (Canning and Mayer, 1966; Allon, 1982; Gortmaker et al., 1993; Enzi, 1994; Gorstein and Grosse, 1994).

It has been argued that obesity is one of the most important preventable causes of ill health and represents a major avoidable contribution to the cost of illness (Kent and Bowyer, 1992; Colditz, 1992) and yet evidence exists to suggest that nutritional problems are on the increase.

Evidence for the effectiveness of preventive measures in nutritional disorders is relatively sparse and, while prevention may be central to the government's strategy to deal with obesity, resistance to changes in lifestyle may make progress in this particular area very challenging (West, 1994b).

Review of studies

The paucity of effectiveness studies is reflected in the range of studies available for review, with no firm evidence existing as to the most effective strategy for preventing or treating problems related to nutritional disorders. One relevant study (Kaplan et al., 1988) has already been included in the section considering studies on exercise, while an earlier study by Kaplan and Davies (1986) concluded that there was no firm experimental literature upon which to assess the potential for improved health care outcomes and reduced costs through educational and nutritional services in diabetes care. This is indicative of the majority of studies reviewed in this section.

Beales, P L and Kopelman, P G (1994) 'Options for the management of obesity', *PharmacoEconomics*, 5 (suppl. 1), 18-32.

Problem definition and objectives of investigation

This was not an economic evaluation but a review of the most effective treatment strategies for early management of obesity.

Study design and setting

The study reviewed the literature to determine strategies that would deliver significant weight reduction (defined as 10% of pre-treatment bodyweight) and maintain the weight reduction for at least 5 years. The treatment options considered were dietary modification, behavioural modification, exercise and physical activity, pharmacotherapy, dental splinting, surgery and alternative methods such as acupuncture.

Approaches to costing

No significant consideration of costs other than a recognition that 'the costs of individual therapies must be weighed against the costs of treating comorbid diseases that are likely to develop as a consequence of obesity' and some comments regarding the financial implications and 'quality-of-life' aspects of some of the strategies.

Approaches to outputs and outcomes

Provided a summary of relative success rates achieved by each of the strategies in treating obesity and commented on their limitations.

Conclusions

Most treatment options would achieve the necessary outcomes (10% weight reduction maintained for a five year period), with varying degrees of cost for moderately obese patients. Few single treatments were able to produce consistent results where the extent of the problem was more severe. It was suggested that multidisciplinary approaches, with continued supervision, were superior to single treatments.

Relevance to health promotion agencies

The obvious implication from this study is that the effectiveness and efficiency of secondary and tertiary prevention measures in a problem area such as obesity remains inconclusive and therefore policies should be directed at primary measures to prevent the problem occurring in the first place.

Ensor, T (1991) 'The evaluation of nutritional problems and policy: an economic approach', *Health Promotion International.* **6, 1, 67-72.**

Problem definition and objectives of investigation

This study argued the case for including economics in the framework for evaluating the implications of nutrition policies from the perspective of social welfare.

Study design and setting

The study was not an economic evaluation *per se* but rather a demonstration of how economics could analyse issues surrounding nutrition policy, such as the demand for nutrition in relation to an individual's consumption patterns and the constraints which may impinge on an appropriate and adequate level of nutrition supply.

Approaches to costing

Included costs within the context of social welfare, referring to direct costs of intervention such as expenditures on health education, and indirect costs such as the social cost to those who consumed a risky product in full knowledge of its consequences, which was no longer available at a low price.

Approaches to outputs and outcomes

Argued that in developing a nutritional policy it is important to examine methods of intervention in the market and compare between tax/benefit procedures or specific measures designed to restrict consumption, supply or the impact of such on third parties.

Conclusions

Expressed the view that 'the main issue to consider in constructing a nutritional policy is increasing social welfare', which may result in conflict with those who would wish to see a restriction of foods considered as harmful and so restricting consumer choice.

Relevance to health promotion agencies

This study emphasises that nutrition policies must be developed from an inter-disciplinary perspective and that health promotion agencies have a role to play in engineering such a process. This is supported by an approach taken by the SUPER-project, which is based on the notion that a 'multi-disciplinary approach and health promotion activities linked to existing social networks on an individual level close to daily life will be more effective than traditional nutrition education' (Vaandrager et al., 1993).

Hutton, J (1994) 'The economics of treating obesity', *PharmacoEconomics,* **5 (suppl. 1), 66-72.**

Problem definition and objectives of investigation

This study was constructed from other contributions to a symposium on the costs of obesity in order to present the economic case for treating the condition.

Study design and setting

The paper provided an overview of the economics of treating obesity, the direct effects of obesity on quality of life, the link between obesity and increased incidence of various diseases, the estimated costs to society of the increased disease burden, the costs and effectiveness of available treatments and finally, brought the information together in assessing the economic case for treating obesity.

Approaches to costing

Discussed the direct costs to the health service as a result of the additional demands placed on the services by obese individuals and the indirect costs, for example, resulting from time off work or not being able to undertake normal activities. This was done from a technical perspective and demonstrated how the economic approach should be adopted rather than actually undertaking an economic evaluation.

Approaches to outputs and outcomes

Relied heavily on the results produced by Beales and Kopelman, with some additional comments offered on the cost implications.

Conclusions

Tentatively explored what may be efficient once more work has been undertaken to establish costs, effectiveness and quality-of-life impact of treatment approaches. For example, the author hinted that behaviour modification may be very cost-effective if successful and that interventionist approaches could also be cost-effective for more serious cases.

As with previous studies there is no firm evidence available to drive policy initiatives in the field of nutrition and it may be that health promotion agencies have a role to play in expanding the research base of appropriate evaluations in nutritional programmes.

Kenkel, D.S (1995) 'Should you eat breakfast? Estimates from health production functions', *Health Economics*, 4, 15-29.

Problem definition and objectives of investigation

The paper aimed to assess the impact of lifestyle choices as determinants of health for adults in the USA. It was not an economic evaluation but nevertheless, provided another insight into how economic techniques might be employed by health promotion agencies in determining priorities.

Study design and setting

An econometric specification based on health production functions was employed. The model was based on the assumption that the current health stock of an individual is based on current additions to or reductions of the health stock based on lifestyles and level of schooling plus other factors which may influence the current stock, for example, past health state, age and sex.

Approaches to costing

No costs were considered in this article.

Approaches to outputs and outcomes

The extent to which lifestyle factors contributed to health status and levels of activity.

Conclusions

The results of this econometric study showed that there was only limited evidence that eating breakfast had important health benefits, while the same applies to snacking between meals. However, the results consistently indicated that excessive weight, cigarette smoking, heavy drinking, excessive or insufficient sleep and stress were harmful inputs in the production of health, while exercise and moderate alcohol consumption emerged as beneficial health inputs.

Relevance to health promotion agencies

The study may point to some refocusing in strategic terms given the dubious nature of eating habits on health status, but it is advocated that a similar investigation be undertaken in the UK context before any firm policy changes are considered.

Strategic developments

The lack of firm evidence is a major problem in developing recommendations for the development of an efficient nutrition strategy. It would appear that, until the research base is expanded, health promotion agencies activities should focus on primary prevention measures related to daily life and be part of broader lifestyle programmes.

10. Safety

Overview

The annual cost to the economy of work-based accidents has been estimated to be between £11 billion and £16 billion per year. This represents between 2-3% of the gross domestic product in the UK or about £200 for every person in the workforce. Accidents at work killed nearly 400 people in 1994, with another 29,000 suffering major injuries such as broken limbs, amputations or severe burns. Other figures from the *Labour Force Survey* (CSO, 1994) suggest that each year nearly one in every 16 people suffers an injury at work and about 17,500 people have to retire prematurely due to work-related ill-health.

While there is evidence that employers are giving a high priority to training in health and safety terms much more is needed to cut down on the two million working days lost per year plus other consequences associated with accidents and injury in the workplace (Schofield, 1995).

However, more accidents occur in the home than in work and injuries are the leading cause of death and a major cause of serious morbidity and disability among children and youth and it has been argued that children's injury prevention is the most deserving case for 'preventionists' attention, since injury typically involved not only physical but economic and psychological disruption for the child, the family and the community' (Peterson et al.,1988).

Review of studies

The literature search provided very few relevant studies for consideration, which reflects, for example, that only a relatively small proportion of mass communication programmes for health and safety have ever been subjected to effectiveness evaluation, and those that have been evaluated lack scientific rigour (Wilde, 1993).

Four studies have been reviewed, two of which look at accidents involving motor vehicles, one which is focused on the prevention of injuries to children and the fourth, which looks at the effectiveness of a scheme designed to reduce the number of falls among the elderly.

Chorba, T L (1991) 'Assessing technologies for preventing injuries in motor vehicle crashes', *International Journal of Technology Assessment in Health Care,* **7, 3, 296-314.**

Problem definition and objectives of investigation

The study examined the effectiveness, use and legislation of safety belts and airbags, using process, injury and economic outcome measures.

Study design and setting

The author employed the *Haddon matrix* as the basis for dividing the sequence of events in crashes into the pre-crash, crash and post-crash phases and the factors that determined the magnitude of each phase. The pre-crash phase included all circumstances that determine whether a crash will occur, for example, driving ability and road conditions; the crash phase included all circumstances that determine whether injury occurs and the nature and severity of injury once the crash occurs, for example, the age and physical condition of the occupants of the vehicle, the size and deformability of the vehicle(s) involved; the post-crash phase included all circumstances that determine the extent to which injury is limited and health restored after the crash, including the time of response by emergency services, subsequent medical care and rehabilitation. The author stated that the *Haddon matrix* has wide application in all areas of injury by providing important determinants of process, injury and economic outcomes to which counter measures can be applied.

Approaches to costing

While recognising that economic outcomes are the most difficult to measure, the author highlighted two of the approaches available for estimating indirect costs (human-capital approach and willingness-to-pay). Estimates of the total economic cost of seat-belt use and crash-associated injuries were included in the study.

Approaches to outputs and outcomes

Considered the process outcomes (changes in belt-use rates, numbers of speeding tickets), injury outcomes (changes in numbers or rates of fatal or disabling injuries) and economic outcomes (cost-benefit evaluations) arising from a variety of measures - seat-belts, airbags, legislation - designed to prevent injuries and disabilities resulting from road traffic accidents.

Conclusions

Argued that 'educational interventions to increase the voluntary use of safety belts, mandatory belt use legislation and the manufacture and installation of automatic belts and airbags can each reduce the indirect costs to society.'

Relevance to health promotion agencies

The *Haddon matrix* may be a useful technique for appraising approaches to be employed across a range of promotional activities, while in specific terms, health promotion agencies can contribute to the promotion of safe driving techniques, knowing that the benefits outweigh the costs of such interventions.

Johnston, I R (1992) 'Traffic safety education: panacea, prophylactic or placebo?', *World Journal of Surgery*, 16, 3, 374-378.

Problem definition and objectives of investigation

The author was of the view that while education is seen as the major strategy for achieving lasting change in traffic safety there was considerable debate as to the effectiveness of such programmes. He presented the case for a more rigorous scientific approach to programme planning and execution and the need for evaluation to be an integral component of such programmes.

Study design and setting

A personal treatise from a surgeon whose aim was to ensure that 'if surgeons are to continue to advocate educational intervention then they should be aware of these issues so that the effectiveness of their efforts is maximised.'

Approaches to costing

Recognition of the role of economic evaluation in determining where resources should be allocated but no explicit attempt to cost any of the policies available for road safety education.

Approaches to outputs and outcomes

Discussed five potential policies for traffic safety measures in terms of the time-frame of their operation, the nature of the causal chain between the measure and the ultimate goal of crash or injury reduction and the degree to which their effectiveness was amenable to scientific evaluation, 'especially cost-benefit analysis.'

Conclusions

Argued that clearly targeted and well designed policies (for example, use of headlights by motorcyclists in daylight) could be cost-effective. In addition, measures which seek to enhance the effectiveness of a second measure (for example, an education programme to increase awareness of an intensive, highly visible random breath-testing operation) could also be shown to be efficient, with the effectiveness able to be compared with other options available for decreasing alcohol-related crashes and the costs of the education programme attached to the other costs in the cost-benefit analysis. Other policies, which aim to create a 'climate of concern' or change social norms or develop general skills and attitudes, were much more difficult to evaluate with scientific rigour. The case was therefore made for such 'lifestyle-change' programmes to compete for resources from the public health field rather than from the traffic safety budget.

Relevance to health promotion agencies

Health promotion agencies have a role to play in reducing the number of road traffic accidents and their consequences and they may be encouraged to work alongside agencies directly involved in road traffic safety at one level, while also pursuing policies which result in lifestyle changes across a number of health threatening and damaging activities.

Peterson, L et al. (1988) 'Community interventions in children's injury prevention: differing costs and differing benefits', *Community Psychology,* **16, 188-204.**

Problem definition and objectives of investigation

The study compared three studies which sought to examine methods available within the community for home safety skill instruction opportunities.

Study design and setting

Two of the studies utilised parents as training agents, one of the reasons being to provide a cost-effective solution to the problem of obtaining a volunteer for each child, while the third study assessed a low-cost hospital-based workshop as a method for improving home skills. Different design strategies were employed for each of the studies.

Approaches to costing

A very basic approach to costing was employed with the assumption that the only actual direct financial costs incurred constituted the cost of the programmes.

Approaches to outputs and outcomes

The series of studies sought to explore ways of preventing injury in the home amongst children particularly vulnerable, in these cases, 'latchkey children' by comparing before and after performance on a number of home safety problem areas.

Conclusions

The results suggested that with hour-long instruction sessions, volunteer parents who received once-weekly professional instruction could effectively teach their children home safety skills across a variety of areas. However, the findings were not replicated across a larger group of parents, whose children volunteered for instruction, due to inadequate instruction by the parents. Similar low-level gains were produced by a hospital-based workshop on home safety.

Relevance to health promotion agencies

The findings highlight the need for health promotion agencies to be proactive in working with their children to promote home safety, although the costs involved may mean that such a policy is not necessarily cost-effective. This investigation produced findings that the low-cost programmes produced low-level gains but did not specifically comment on the costs of producing the high-level gains achieved by the first study. The relative efficiency is therefore unproved.

Wagner, E H et al. (1994) 'Preventing disability and falls in older adults: a population-based randomised trial', *American Journal of Public Health,* **84, 11, 1800-1806.**

Problem definition and objectives of investigation

This study reported on a 'modest preventive intervention targeting risk factors for disability and falls among non-disabled older health maintenance organisation enrolees.'

Study design and setting

The study was not an economic evaluation but explored issues which could be taken up by a subsequent economic appraisal.

Approaches to costing

No costs were included, although it would have been possible to include estimates of the cost of nurse visits and follow-up interventions

Approaches to outputs and outcomes

Functional status and incidence of falls were used as the outcomes in the study.

Conclusions

The study showed that the group who received a disability and fall prevention nurse visit plus follow-up interventions reported a significantly lower incidence of declining functional status and a significantly lower incidence of falls than the group who received only the usual care package. Those who received only a nurse visit had intermediate levels of most outcomes. After two years the differentials between the groups narrowed and led the authors to conclude that 'intensifying and sustaining the intervention without making costs prohibitively expensive for public health will be a challenge for future research in this area.'

Relevance to health promotion agencies

Preventive measures have some short-term impact but it is apparent that for this particular segment of the population the medium and long term effects are less convincing. Health promotion agencies could liaise with other agencies in this sphere of activity but there does not appear to be any significant advantage from diverting substantial resources into these activities.

Strategic developments

The lack of effectiveness measures in this area inhibit the extent to which value-for-money approaches can be suggested. However, there is some evidence that primary prevention measures, for example, safe-driving techniques, may prove to be relatively efficient, especially when the messages form part of a collaborative approach from a variety of relevant organisations. There is also evidence that targeting of particular groups may be successful, especially with 'reinforcing messages,' but messages which aim to 'create concern' can be potentially damaging.

The over-riding recommendation here is that, until the research evidence proves otherwise, low-cost measures which generate small scale benefits would appear to be the aim of strategic developments in the area of accident prevention.

11. Sexuality

Overview

Promoting sexual health: the best way to tackle HIV was the title attached to a report on a meeting held in July 1992 'to revitalise the campaign against HIV infection' (Smith, 1992). While sexual health is associated with a range of infections and diseases, the term has become inextricably linked with AIDS and HIV infection. The full extent of the HIV epidemic is unknown and subject to considerable discussion and debate (for example, Hall, 1994; Main, 1993; Piot, 1991; Winn and Skelton, 1992), while the economic impact of AIDS and HIV infection is also the subject of much contemplation in the literature (for example, Andulis and Weslowski, 1992; Drummond and Davies, 1990; Lambert and Carrin, 1990; Lynn et al., 1992; Tolley and Gyldmark, 1993). Some fifteen years after the first cases of AIDS were reported the extent of the problem will present professionals, researchers and policy makers with 'the greatest definitive challenge of the 1990s' (Ting and Carter, 1992), as efforts continue to discover a vaccine or effective cure and preventive schemes seek to diminish the spread of the problem. Preventive measures focus on the risk factors which may result in HIV infection such as drug abuse and sexual practices.

However, while knowledge and attitudes may have changed as a result of the health education messages, this has not been translated into behavioural change and there may have to be considerable political and social change in Britain if the nation's attitude towards sexual behaviour is to be more open and positive (Smith, 1992). This message is a major indictment on the approach of government and others, who argue that receipt of the message will result in behaviour change. For example, the expenditure of £22.5 million by the Department of Health on its advertising campaign during 1986/87 was regarded as the only method of curtailing the spread of the epidemic and yet the evidence that it achieved anything of note is weak, at best (Ross et al., 1989; Wells, 1988). On a wider scale there is fairly conclusive evidence to suggest that mass media campaigns are not very effective agents of change (Redman et al., 1990).

Review of studies

While a number of studies exist which explore the economic consequences of AIDS and HIV infection (for example, Andulis, 1992; Bloom and Glied, 1989; Drummond and Davies (eds), 1990; Morton et al., 1993; Lynn, 1992; Schwefel et al. (eds), 1990; Scitovsky, 1989; Tolley and Gyldmark, 1993), the lack of reliable evidence on the effectiveness of alternative health promotion practices for promoting sexual health as a means of curtailing the AIDS epidemic (Godfrey et al., 1992) has not enabled much work to be undertaken to establish which are the most efficient ways of allocating resources within prevention programmes, which aim at reducing the prevalence of serious health problems associated with sexual practices.

Five studies are included in this section to highlight how economic evaluation can contribute to decisions relating to strategic developments in promoting sexual health.

Godfrey, C and Tolley, K (1992) 'An economic approach to the evaluation of HIV/AIDS health education programmes', in Aggleton, P et al. (eds) *Does it work? perspectives of the evaluation of HIV/AIDS health promotion*, Health Education Authority, London.

Problem definition and objectives of investigation

This paper examined the issues which arise in seeking to apply economic principles to the evaluation of programmes of HIV/AIDS education.

Study design and setting

Discussed the basic principles of economic appraisal and then applied them to HIV/AIDS education programmes.

Approaches to costing

Identified the direct costs which may accrue in a programme and highlighted the need to adopt the *opportunity cost* perspective. Considered the difficulties arising from inter-agency initiatives and where resources, capital and labour, were shared between a number of programmes. Recommended the inclusion of indirect costs, even where measurement and valuation was difficult.

Approaches to outputs and outcomes

Argued for the separation of process from outputs and outcomes in the evaluation of such programmes. Considered the debate as to what constitutes output and outcomes from a health education programme and made reference to the Oxford Regional Health Authority's policy document which sets out targets, which could be measured as an indicator of effectiveness. Also recommended the inclusion of savings in health costs, life years and quality of life considerations within the flow of benefits together with the negative benefits, such as the number of worried well (who emerged as a result of the first mass media campaign) which may result from the programme.

Conclusions

Recognised the difficulties involved in relating changes in behaviour and other benefits to specific programmes and argued that considerable research effort, undertaken centrally, is needed to provide reliable estimates of risk behaviour and to develop scenario analyses.

Relevance to health promotion agencies

Provides a useful framework, within which programmes can be evaluated to assess the extent to which they represent value for money.

Lagergren, M (1990) 'The economic analysis of prevention of HIV infection: evaluation of programmes and decision support for priority setting in health policy - case study Sweden', in Schwefel, D et al. (eds) *Economic aspects of AIDS and HIV* **infection, Springer-Verlag, Berlin.**

Problem definition and objectives of investigation

The study examined the effects of preventive measures on the spread of the AIDS epidemic by utilising a series of 'HIV epidemiological computer models.' Acknowledged that if prevention is to be efficient it will need to employ a range of measures but that each measure should be subjected to evaluation, including an economic component.

Study design and setting

The investigation was based on the theory that in order to prevent an epidemic breaking out necessitated controlling 'the basic reproduction rate' (the product of the number of partners, the probability of transmission per partner and the duration time of infectiousness) so that it stays less than one. Suggested that the goals of prevention may be to reduce the number of contacts with (potentially) infected partners and to reduce the probability of transmission of the virus.

Approaches to costing

Proposed that 'costs' should be interpreted in the broadest sense and include direct and indirect costs but also political and ethical considerations.

Approaches to outputs and outcomes

Recognised the difficulties attached to assessing the benefits of HIV prevention in that data concerning infectivity, rate of contacts and partner change, relationships between different groups, etc. are extremely unlikely to be available, thus preventing 'precise cost benefit evaluations' to be undertaken.

Offered reduced number of deaths in a specific time period as one possible outcome measure, and tested the impact of preventive measures in securing such an outcome against certain assumptions.

Conclusions

Examined the impact of screening certain proportions of the high-risk population and showed that if 30% in the group are screened and 50% of those with HIV stop spreading the disease the number of deaths in 20 years would be reduced by 50%. However, the effect would not be as favourable over a longer period of time because the basic reproduction rate would not have fallen below 1 and hence the epidemic would have been postponed rather than inhibited.

The study also examined the impact of condom use in reducing the transmission risk in a high risk and a low risk group. Showed that 75% condom usage in the high risk group would postpone the epidemic but such use in the low risk group would cause the prevalence of HIV infection to decrease over time. Concluded that preventive strategies must be directed towards halting the spread within groups at high risk and reducing the number of infections that these groups may pass to other groups.

Relevance to health promotion agencies

The last sentence in this article reads 'the problem is to maintain efforts in the long run when the public arousal triggered by the first appearance of the epidemic has subsided.' It is here where health promotion agencies have a role. The most efficient strategy provided by the computer model is one where there is a reduction in partner frequency both within and outside the low risk group. Health promotion agencies should therefore seek to encourage such moves.

Ohi, G et al. (1987) 'AIDS prevention in Japan and its cost-benefit aspects,' *Health Policy*, 8, 17-27.

Problem definition and objectives of investigation

The study aimed to undertake an economic analysis of public health programmes designed to counter the spread of AIDS in Japan and estimate the future incidence of the disease.

Study design and setting

Estimates of the incidence of the disease were based on a Delphi exercise in a country where the population of homosexual men and drug abusers are 'far smaller than those in the USA.' Economic analyses were based on the projected incidence of AIDS.

Approaches to costing

Estimated the costs of a number of programmes categorised into education and surveillance and provision of safe blood-supply and blood-donor screening.

Approaches to outputs and outcomes

Identified the direct benefits as savings of medical costs for the diagnosis and treatment of AIDS patients and the value of productivity loss saved as the indirect benefits resulting from the programmes.

Conclusions

The results of the 'cost-benefit' analysis was dependent on the scale of the blood donor screening programme. Programmes focused on counselling were shown to be highly cost-effective (the programmes would be justified on economic grounds if only two cases were prevented) but screening of all blood donors in metropolitan areas would yield a net loss given estimates of the impact of the disease in Japan.

Relevance to health promotion agencies

Very different socio-economic factors exist in Japan to UK but it does provide evidence that careful targeting and counselling of high risk groups can be a very efficient approach to generating health gain.

The claim that screening of blood donors was not cost effective and should perhaps not form part of a prevention policy was questioned by Lee and Moss (1987). They argue that policies must be 'culturally appropriate' if they are to be effective and lend weight to the argument that economic appraisal can only form part of the decision making process in determining policy directions.

Rovira, J (1990) 'Economics of prevention', in Drummond M F and Davies, L (eds) *AIDS: the challenge for economic analysis*, Health Service Management Centre, University of Birmingham.

Problem definition and objectives of investigation

This paper was an economic appraisal of AIDS preventive measures.

Study design and setting

Commenced from the premise that while policies directed at the high risk groups may be the most effective this may not always be the case and examined the relative efficiency of measures designed to screen for AIDS and health education programmes .

Approaches to costing

Did not pay much attention to costs arguing that 'the measurement and estimation of the costs of programmes to prevent AIDS do not seem to pose particular problems for economic evaluation.'

Approaches to outputs and outcomes

Concentrated on the benefits side of the appraisal and suggested that benefits should be related to the approach adopted for the economic evaluation, and consist of savings in healthcare resources, QALYs, productivity gains, etc.

Debated how some of these could be considered within an AIDS setting and the role of 'intangibles', such as reduction of anxiety and fear.

Conclusions

Concluded that economic evaluation was useful in determining the optimal alternative in very specific decision problems and in considering which groups should be targeted with health promotion messages.

Relevance to health promotion agencies

The major message from this paper is that targeting is, in general. effective but that other factors have to be brought into the decision making arena. For example, if the future spread of AIDS is likely to be dependent on heterosexual transmission, then there is a strong case for placing resources into programmes designed to minimise the impact of a multiplicity of sexual partners rather than focusing on high risk groups, especially amongst those who may be reluctant to accept any external intervention.

Soderlund, N et al. (1993) 'The costs of HIV prevention strategies in developing countries', *Bulletin of the World Health Organisation*, 71, 5, 595-604.

Problem definition and objectives of investigation

The article reported on a preliminary attempt to assess the costs and outputs of a sample of HIV prevention strategies, namely, mass media campaigns, peer education programmes, sexually transmitted disease treatment, condom social marketing, safe blood provision and needle exchange/bleach provision programmes.

Study design and setting

Utilised data from published studies or directly from project co-ordinators. The setting for all studies was within developing countries.

Approaches to costing

Costs were classified into capital costs and recurrent costs, which were further subdivided into salaries and other costs.

Approaches to outputs and outcomes

Very crude indicators of output were used, for example, teachers trained, condoms distributed, number of visits, number of contacts, and the authors refer to them as process measures.

Conclusions

Findings suggested that condom social marketing projects were less costly than condom distribution programmes but this approach may not be as effective in reaching vulnerable groups. Person to person peer education programmes were more expensive per contact than school education programmes but again they may be more effective in reaching high risk groups.

Recognition of the methodological flaws in the data collection and analysis but presented a clear agenda for future research in the economic evaluation of HIV prevention strategies.

Relevance to health promotion agencies

Confirms that targeting of the groups most at risk is seen as a cost-effective strategy in promoting sexual health, while doubts are again expressed, though not explicitly, of the wisdom of mass campaigns in the media.

Strategic developments

There is reasonable evidence to suggest that measures designed to reduce the number of sexual partners are efficient. There is less clear evidence as to whether there should be specific targeting of high risk groups with such measures, while the effectiveness for screening is dubious while mass media campaigns are probably ineffective, especially if the 'scare factor' is incorporated.

Health promotion agencies should therefore concentrate attention on efficient policies designed to promote 'healthy sexuality' with minimum partners and the use of condoms.

12. Smoking

Overview

Smoking is widely acknowledged as one of the largest single causes of premature death and preventable ill health and it has been suggested that eliminating smoking would increase population-wide life expectancy by approximately 1 year (Tsevat, 1992). Evidence now suggests that smoking contributes to over 20 diseases and that a quarter of those who smoke cigarettes regularly will eventually be killed as a result of their 'health damaging' behaviour, and that prolonged smoking increases 3-fold the risk of premature death in middle age and that about 50% of all long term cigarette smokers die early (Doll, 1993).

The impact of smoking, and other health damaging behaviours, imposes costs at the individual level, e.g. costs of purchasing the cigarettes and the increased risk of illness and premature death, but also for society as a whole, in the form of, for example, the increased risks from passive smoking, fire risks and environmental damage. Estimates of the medical costs of smoking range from $US54 per smoker per year to $US1,058 per smoker per year (1990 prices) (Phillips, 1993). However, the vast range of estimated costs highlights the need for caution in its interpretation. In the UK context, it has been estimated that the annual smoking cost to NHS hospitals was over £350 million (1990-91 prices) (Mawhinney, 1993); that the number of working days lost in the UK range between 16 million and over 50 million days (Cohen, 1984; Royal College of Physicians, 1977) ; in Wales the estimate of costs to the NHS was nearly £26 million (Health Education Authority, 1991) and the number of working days lost annually was estimated at being in excess of 1.2 million (although this study only considered the effects of smoking on lung cancer, coronary heart disease and chronic bronchitis) (Phillips and Prowle, 1993).

While there is evidence of a decline in smoking (Chapman, 1992), there are a number of causes for concern. These include the proportion of children smoking and some evidence from the US that smoking decline has plateaued after two decades. health promotion agencies, together with other organisations, remain committed to achieving a 20% reduction in the level of smoking by the year 2000. However, achievement of targets by the year 2000 will 'require rapid implementation of cost-effective interventions with a major impact both on public policy - for example, cigarette taxation - and on the behaviour of large numbers of smokers. Interventions in this category include mass communications and opportunistic advice from the family doctor' (Reid et al., 1992). In addition, recent reviews have highlighted that tobacco use constitutes the single largest threat to the health of the nation (Bartecchi et al., 1993; MacKenzie et al., 1994; Doll et al., 1994).

Review of studies

The literature review has revealed a number of studies examining the economic aspects of smoking cessation programmes, although the number is small relative to the number of studies on the effectiveness of such programmes. However, there is concern over the general lack of quality displayed in the investigations (Elixhauser, 1990; Cohen and Fowler, 1993) and problems exist in seeking to replicate the studies in other contexts. What is not in debate is that 'interventions aimed at getting smokers to quit are among the most cost-effective uses of healthcare resources' (Tsevat, 1992).

The studies highlighted below concentrate on those areas which are of more direct relevance to health promotion agencies and therefore, studies which relate to advice from GPs to quit smoking (for example, Williams, 1987; Cummings et al., 1989) and studies which evaluate the use of nicotine gum as an adjunct to counselling from doctors (for example, Tsevat, 1992) have not been included. The evidence on the cost effectiveness of nicotine gum is sensitive to the setting of the investigation - the same degree of success has not been demonstrated in general practice as that achieved in specialist clinics (Hughes et al., 1989; Hjalmarson, 1984) and should be the subject of further investigations. No economic evaluations of nicotine patches and nicotine nasal spray and inhaler (Sutherland et al., 1992) were discovered, and should therefore be included in the research agenda for the efficiency of smoking cessation programmes.

In undertaking the literature search for health promotion activities designed to reduce smoking, two literature reviews (Elixhauser, 1990; Cohen and Fowler, 1993) were utilised as part of the process in addition to the on-line searches undertaken.

As with other areas there is evidence that specific targeting of health promotion increases the extent of the benefits produced. The first study to be reviewed is one examining the relative efficiency of a programme designed at reducing smoking amongst pregnant women. The benefits to pregnant women from a cessation in smoking (reduced risk of low birthweight, ontrauterine growth retardation and perinatal mortality) will result in an enhanced stream of benefits which will, in all probability, result in schemes aimed at such a group being more cost-beneficial than those aimed at the general population.

Marks, J S, et al. (1990) 'A cost-benefit/cost-effectiveness analysis of smoking cessation for pregnant women', *American Journal of Preventive Medicine,* **6, 5, 282-289.**

Problem definition and objectives of investigation

The study estimated the cost-effectiveness of a smoking cessation programme for pregnant women designed to reduce low birthweight and perinatal mortality. The question posed at the outset of this investigation was 'what would be the projected costs and outcomes if all pregnant women who smoked cigarettes took part in a smoking cessation program early in their pregnancy?'

Study design and setting

The study was, in effect, a model which consisted of a counselling session, instructional materials and two follow-up telephone calls. Smoking and cessation rates were estimated from previous studies which enabled predictions to be made of the differences between smokers and non-smokers in the number of low birthweight infants and the number of perinatal deaths.

Approaches to costing

Direct costs involved in the programme were included - staff time for telephone conversations, cost of materials, plus overheads to cover staff training - and estimated to amount to $30 per participant, although a range of costs from $5 to $100 were used as part of the sensitivity analysis. No indirect costs were included, the argument being that follow-on visits were part of routine care.

Approaches to outputs and outcomes

The outcomes were expressed in terms of costs averted (that is, costs per average birth for hospitalisation low birthweight infants minus those costs for normal birthweight infants) plus estimates savings accruing from reductions in excessive impairments and associated care for low birthweight infants with conditions such as cerebral palsy, mental retardation or both. No consideration was given to the savings generated by women who quit due to fewer maternal complications or chronic conditions and the lifetime earnings of infants whose deaths would be prevented. Sensitivity analysis was also applied to the measurement of outcomes, by varying the quit rates, the proportion of low birthweight infants requiring neonatal intensive care, the relative risk of having a low birthweight infant and of perinatal death.

Conclusions

If the hypothetical programme were applied to all pregnant women who smoke in the USA it was estimated that it would cost $4,000 per low birthweight birth prevented, $2,934 per life year gained (using a discount factor of 4%) and save $3.31 in neonatal intensive care costs plus $3.26 from prevented disability for every $1 spent on the programme. The results of the sensitivity analysis produced a cost for each low birthweight birth prevented of $13,333 when the cost of the programme was $100 per participant, if the quit rate was 5%, rather than the 15% employed, the cost would be $12,000. The authors demonstrated that the benefit to cost ratio of 6.6:1 was impressive when compared to other studies, for example, neonatal metabolic screening, screening for Down's syndrome in women over 40 and prenatal care, even when more stringent assumptions are built into the analysis.

Relevance to health promotion agencies

While recognising the need for caution in interpreting benefit to cost ratios, which the authors acknowledge, it does provide health promotion agencies with very useful information, supported by other studies from the USA (Ershoff et al., 1990; Shipp et al., 1992; Windsor et al., 1993) with which to emphasise the attractiveness of investing in programmes designed to minimise smoking amongst pregnant women. The authors conclude that '...public health programs should offer this preventive service to all pregnant women who smoke.'

Tillgren, P et al. (1993) 'Cost-effectiveness of a tobacco "Quit and Win" contest in Sweden', *Health Policy,* **26, 43-53.**

Problem definition and objectives of investigation

The explicit aim of this study was to 'present an analysis of the Stockholm Quit and Win contest and to discuss the methodological potential and limitations of such an analysis.'

Study design and setting

The Quit and Win contest, a collaborative venture involving a number of organisations, in and around Stockholm, was aimed at participants aged 16 and over who had used tobacco daily for at least twelve months and at 'recruiters,' who were to enrol friends or members of their family into the contest. The campaign commenced with a 3-week recruitment period before 'Quit Day' when participants were to stop using tobacco. They had to abstain from all kinds of tobacco for four weeks, could not resort to smoking cessation aids containing nicotine and then had to pass a cotton test to verify their abstinence.

Approaches to costing

The direct costs of the programme and its evaluation were used. The 'personnel costs' were based on responses to enquiries made to the project group and collaborating organisations in which they estimated number of people, time spent and salary for each person involved in the programme. No indirect costs were included.

Approaches to outputs and outcomes

The main outcome indicator was years of life saved (YLS). Data relating to changes in use of tobacco was based on the entry forms and two different random samples at 6 months and 12 months after the contest. The effects of the contest were estimated as the number of participants who were non-smoking after 12 months less the number of spontaneous smokers (those who during the same time period had quit, irrespective of the contest).

Conclusions

The costs per YLS of the contest varied from $160 to $2,450 depending upon the assumptions, which the authors argue is cost-effective in comparison to other medical interventions, a view they support with reference to other studies

(Oster et al., 1986; Williams, 1987; Cummings et al., 1989). However, in a study to assess the cost-effectiveness of three smoking cessation programmes, the contest was more cost-effective than a smoking cessation class but less cost-effective than a self-help programme (Altman et al., 1987). Such findings led the authors to conclude that combining cessation programmes may lead to an increase in effectiveness, arguing that 'different smoking cessation programs may attract different types of people and preferences for cessation programs may shift over time.' The Swedish study also offered similar advice and showed that the effects were much more pronounced when both the mass media strategy was combined with an organisation strategy. However, the major problem with this type of study lies in seeking to control for the effects of the 'intervention', an issue which was also pertinent in the next study reviewed.

Relevance to health promotion agencies

There is no doubt that contests are relatively cost-effective although the extent of their effectiveness depends largely on the quit rate achieved and, as the proportion of the population who smoke decreases, the extent to which such strategies are effective may also decline, given that the smoking population may be less inclined to 'kick the habit'. It may be advisable, therefore, to collect more extensive data on the differential attraction of smoking cessation programmes for sub-groups within the population.

Phillips, C J and Prowle, M J (1993) 'Economics of a reduction in smoking: case study from Heartbeat Wales', *Journal of Epidemiology and Community Health,* **47, 215-223.**

Problem definition and objectives of investigation

The study aimed to assess the costs and benefits of the Heartbeat Wales No-Smoking Intervention Programme, which itself had sought to reduce smoking prevalence within the Principality by 1% per year for the period 1985-90.

Study design and setting

The study examined the costs and benefits to the health service as one aspect and a broader economic appraisal. where the costs and benefits to industry and commerce were also included. Data relating to smoking prevalence was acquired from population surveys undertaken in 1985 and 1988, which demonstrated that there was an overall decline in smoking prevalence in Wales of 4.1% in men and 2.7% in women, which more or less complied with the target set by Heartbeat Wales in its planning document.

Approaches to costing

The authors admitted to employing a pragmatic approach to costing, including those costs 'which can be estimated with reasonable objectivity' but 'in other cases the existence of such costs has merely been noted'. The direct costs of activities relating to the programme were included from organisations involved (Health Promotion Authority for Wales, district health authorities and industry and commerce) but no quantification of indirect costs was undertaken, although the sensitivity analysis sought to 'compensate' for their omission.

Approaches to outputs and outcomes

The study distinguished between the intermediate outcome, that is the reduction in smoking prevalence, and final outcomes, identified as reduced morbidity, displaced mortality and environmental changes and expressed as benefits to the NHS, benefits to employers, benefits to the individual and benefits to society. The impact of reduced smoking prevalence was concentrated on three disease categories - coronary heart disease, lung cancer and bronchial disease - with timing profiles applied to identify when the risk factors were eliminated. Benefits were measured in monetary terms and in life years saved.

Conclusions

To counter the difficulty of determining the effect of the intervention a series of 'impact rates' were utilised to assess the cost-benefit and cost-utility of the programme. The results showed that if Heartbeat Wales was 'responsible' for 10% of the reduction in smoking prevalence in Wales there were substantial net monetary benefits of nearly £4 million and the cost per working life year saved was £58. Downward adjustments to the stream of benefits and altering the timing profiles so that the reduction in risks were delayed still produced significant net monetary benefits of over £2.5 million and a cost per working life year saved of £64.

Relevance to health promotion agencies

The study was an evaluation of the programme during the first few years of its inception. As stated above the impact of smoking cessation programmes changes over time and the proportion of smokers who remain are the 'hard core' who are less responsive to the health promotion messages. Linking health promotion messages to fiscal measures may increase the extent of the decline in smoking (Townsend, 1987; Hu et al., 1995). Evidence also suggests that smoking occurs in the context of an overall health behaviour pattern, which includes excessive drinking and physical inactivity and that policies might 'become more effective by broadening their focus to address health behaviour patterns, rather than single risk behaviours' (Hu et al., 1995).

Haycox, A (1994) 'A methodology for estimating the costs and benefits of health promotion', *Health Promotion International.* 9, 1, 5-11.

Problem definition and objectives of investigation

The study described an alternative evaluative methodology to demonstrate the benefits that can be derived from health promotion schemes by quantifying the direct impact of health promotion on health gain and resource use.

Study design and setting

The study utilised a simulation model based on current life-tables to estimate the cost implications arising from any health promotion programme and the life years gained by the programme. The case study used for the analysis was a health promotion programme aimed at reducing smoking behaviour by the population served within the North West Regional Health Authority.

Approaches to costing

The study focused on the resource impact of the health promotion campaign in the short-term, by examining the costs involved in funding the programme; in the medium-term, by considering the resource savings to the health service as a consequence of reductions in smoking related illnesses; and in the long-term, by highlighting the increased demand for health service resources from a larger elderly population as a consequence of reductions in smoking related mortality.

Approaches to outputs and outcomes

The author took the current 'stock' of residents within the region and projected their likely mortality experience until no one remained on the basis of current mortality trends. The mortality experience was altered by the health promotion programme and a different profile emerged which enabled the additional number of life years to be gauged.

Conclusions

The hypothetical programme would lead to a 0.15% increase in the total life years within the region, which was then translated into resource implications for the health service. While there would be an increase in hospital and community costs they would be more than offset by a reduction in primary care costs. The effect of discounting (by 6%) both life years gained and costs the programme were estimated to produce a cost *decrease* of £301 (males) and £402 (females). The author adds, 'there can surely be few health care interventions that simultaneously offer such significant health care benefits and resource savings.'

Relevance to health promotion agencies

This study claims to offer an 'extremely flexible framework by which to quantify the overall costs and benefits arising from health promotion campaigns' by enabling the 'user' to alter the assumptions used based on perceptions and improved data. As with previous studies it confirms the efficiency of programmes designed to reduce smoking prevalence but also could be used to compare programme in terms of their relative efficiency. The basic problem with all studies lies in determining the extent to which the effects can be attributed to the intervention and also the extent to which the behaviour contributes to the disease. Much more work is needed of an epidemiological nature to enable economic evaluations to be anything other than reasonable guestimates of the efficiency of health promotion programmes.

Strategic developments

Most work on the efficiency of health promotion measures has been undertaken in this area and therefore the scope for development of policies which will maximise returns on investment is also more evident in this area of activity.

The literature demonstrates that where smoking cessation programmes can be 'bolted-on' to other interventions there are obvious attractions, for example, programmes with pregnant women receiving prenatal care. Obviously, those measures which maximise quit rates are likely to be more efficient although some concerns are expressed that schemes which have proved to be effective and efficient in recent times, may suffer from a declining percentage of willing quitters in the population, and be less successful in the future. On-going monitoring and evaluation of successful programmes needs to be in place to ensure that resources are continued to be directed in the most appropriate direction.

In addition, there is evidence to support the view that health promotion should be linked and supported by stronger taxation measures to make it less attractive in financial, as well as health, terms to continue to smoke.

13. Conclusions

Health policy issues are high on the political agendas of all countries and are likely to remain so. The advancements in technological developments and medical science coupled with the increasing expectations of communities as to what is available from health care providers continue to focus attention on the health care dilemma. This book has aimed to show how the utilisation of economic techniques can identify health promotion interventions which will provide value for money and which will assist in maximising the health care benefits generated by the resource available. The nature of the health care dilemma and, more generally the basic economic problem, means that choices will always have to be made as to the level of resources allocated to health care and, within health care, which areas are to receive a greater share and which areas should receive less. In making such choices there is a need for an explicit set of priorities to be established. The discipline of economics can play a major role in fulfilling this need. Traditional approaches have been shown to be of limited validity and avoid consideration of the fact that resources used in one area on one programme are not available for other programmes or for use in other areas.

The literature survey demonstrated that in the majority of areas of health promotion activities, there were very few studies which had incorporated a clear economic perspective and on which firm conclusions could be reached as to the directions and policies health promotion should focus. The major problem surrounded what health promotion was seeking to accomplish. The outcomes of health promotion are still far from clearly defined and this, coupled with the uncertainty as to whether health promotion is effective in securing behaviour change, as opposed to changes in knowledge and awareness, has acted as a severe constraint on schemes being subjected to economic evaluation.

The use of data relating to the costs of certain diseases to the health service and to society is a popular approach for estimating the impact of health promotion in reducing risk factors associated with such diseases. However, reliance on such approaches may lead to the mistaken view that health promotion should be increasingly used as a vehicle for reducing the financial pressures on the health service and public services in general. It must be stressed that health promotion and participation in health promotion activities is not costless and in considering the value for money secured by health promotion a broad view of efficiency, looking at both sides of the efficiency coin, needs to be adopted. The aim must be that whatever resources are allocated to health promotion they should be utilised so as to secure the maximum impact for society in terms of improved health status, freeing up resources in other sectors of the health service, economic performance as well as the financial incentives. There are clear procedures to adopt in undertaking economic evaluations and they should be used so that all costs and all benefits of the programme are at the very least identified and, as large a proportion as feasible, quantified and valued in terms of health status or quasi-monetary indicators.

With regard to the length of time it takes for health promotion activities to generate benefits the issue of discounting is particularly relevant. The debate is ongoing in the literature but whereas there are strong grounds for discounting financial benefits, the case for discounting health improvements is much less clear cut. It is essential that sensitivity analysis is employed to demonstrate the effect of using varying rates of discount and present the complete information picture to decision makers.

The review of the literature did produce some broad perspectives on the potential directions for health promotion agencies' strategic developments but they need to be subjected to further detailed investigation, including an economic assessment, before any clear impressions can be gained. In addition, the replication of programmes and policies which have been tried and tested in one community or country may not be applicable in other communities and cultures. The cultural dimension is one which should not be neglected in determining policy and it also provides weight to the argument that evaluation of policies and programmes should encompass a suitable criterion to assess the suitability of programmes for specific communities and cultures.

Another message which comes across from all areas of activity is that, in general, targeting of programmes and policies is likely to be more effective in securing health gain. There are negative features to be considered as well, however, in that a large proportion of those who are unlikely to take heed of the health promotion messages may actually form the composition of the high risk groups. More research is needed to test this hypothesis, which alongside the cultural dimension should find itself high up on the research agenda for health education and health promotion.

There are clearly areas where the effectiveness of health promotion and prevention is not questioned and in these areas this has been translated into a demonstration of the efficiency of allocating resources to programmes in these areas. However, in other areas the causal relationships are more dubious and more research is needed to establish the links, and the nature and strength of such links, between preventive measures and behaviour change.

One potential solution is to ensure that strategies have a wide focus and are not 'area-specific'. The literature clearly demonstrates that programmes which seek to address more than one risk factor are likely to be more effective than measures which are highly specific. Programmes which aim to demonstrate the dangers and disadvantages to individuals, identified as being in high risk groups, of 'inappropriate' lifestyles (and the implications for other members of their families and community) may be the most efficient direction for health promotion agencies to move in the short-term at least. This could be accompanied by on-going liaison with other organisations (employers, unions, community associations, churches, etc.) in an attempt to disperse the costs and ensure that for health promotion agencies, there will be returns on their investment.

Therefore, in seeking to assist decision-makers in the field of health promotion, a series of recommendations arising from the literature and based on the economic framework surrounding the review are proposed. They are:

- To continue to engage in research to determine the outcomes generated by health promotion which can be utilised in economic evaluation of programmes.

- To move towards a priority based approach in constructing health promotion initiatives so that maximum health benefits can be generated.

- To employ appropriate techniques when undertaking economic appraisals and not rely on cost-of-illness approaches.

- To incorporate sensitivity analysis in the economic appraisals to allow for costs and benefits not quantified and valued.

- To discount monetary benefits arising from health promotion programmes at the prevailing rate but to use a reduced or zero rate in discounting health benefits (and using sensitivity analysis to highlight implications).

- To liaise with relevant organisations in providing activities to avoid artificial settings but also to disperse the costs involved.

- To focus on activities where effectiveness and efficiency have been clearly demonstrated and facilitate research in other areas to improve knowledge and research base.

- To target the campaigns where maximum impact will be achieved, having regard for likely response and probability of behaviour change.

- To ensure that programmes and policies are 'culture specific.'

- To establish a pluralistic evaluation framework for programmes which would include efficiency as one of a number of criteria.

Bibliography

Studies reviewed

Albee, G (1994) 'The fourth revolution' in Trent, D R and Reed, C *Promotion of mental health: Volume 3-1993*, Avebury, Aldershot.

Beales, P L and Kopelman, P G (1994) 'Options for the management of obesity', *PharmacoEconomics*, 5 (suppl. 1), pp. 18-32.

Burton, W N (1991) 'Value-managed mental health benefits', *Journal of Occupational Medicine*, 33, 3, pp. 311-313.

Chorba, T L (1991) 'Assessing technologies for preventing injuries in motor vehicle crashes', *International Journal of Technology Assessment in Health Care*, 7, 3, pp. 296-314.

Ensor, T (1991) 'The evaluation of nutritional problems and policy: an economic approach', *Health Promotion International.* 6, 1, pp. 67-72.

Godfrey, C (1994) 'Assessing the cost-effectiveness of alcohol services', *Journal of Mental Health*, 3, pp. 3-21.

Godfrey, C and Tolley, K (1992) 'An economic approach to the evaluation of HIV/AIDS health education programmes', in Aggleton, P et al. (eds) *Does it work? perspectives of the valuation of HIV/AIDS health promotion*, Health Education Authority, London.

Hatziandreu, E I et al. (1988) 'A cost-effectiveness analysis of exercise as a health promotion activity', *American Journal of Public Health*, 78, 11, pp. 1417-1421.

Haycox, A (1994) 'A methodology for estimating the costs and benefits of health promotion', *Health Promotion International,* 9, 1, pp. 5-11.

Hobson, S and Cameron, I (1994) 'Feeling good in Burley: Evaluation of a week to promote mental health', in Trent, D R and Reed, C *Promotion of mental health: Volume 3-1993*, Avebury, Aldershot.

Hutton, J (1994) 'The economics of treating obesity', PharmacoEconomics, 5 (suppl. 1), pp. 66-72.

Johnston, I R (1992) 'Traffic safety education: panacea, prophylactic or placebo?' World Journal of Surgery, 16, 3, pp. 374-378.

Kaplan, R M et al. (1988) 'The cost-utility of diet and exercise interventions in non-insulin dependent diabetes mellitus', Health Promotion, 2, 4, pp. 331-340.

Kenkel, D S (1995) 'Should you eat breakfast? Estimates from health production functions', Health Economics, 4, pp. 15-29.

Lagergren, M (1990) 'The economic analysis of prevention of HIV infection: evaluation of programmes and decision support for priority setting in health policy-case study Sweden,' in Schwefel, D et al. (eds) Economic aspects of AIDS and HIV infection, Springer-Verlag, Berlin.

Light, D and Bailey, V (1993) 'Pound foolish', Health Service Journal. 11 February, pp. 16-18.

Marks, J S, et al. (1990) 'A cost-benefit/cost-effectiveness analysis of smoking cessation for pregnant women', American Journal of Preventive Medicine, 6, 5, pp. 282-289.

Maynard, A and Godfrey, C (1994) 'Alcohol policy - evaluating the options', British Medical Bulletin, 50, 1, pp. 221-230.

Nicholl, J P et al. (1994) 'Health and health care costs and benefits of exercise', PharmacoEconomics, 5, 2, pp. 109-122.

Ohi, G et al. (1987) 'AIDS prevention in Japan and its cost-benefit aspects', Health Policy, 8, pp. 17-27.

Orlandi, M A et al. (1990) 'Computer-assisted strategies for substance abuse prevention: opportunities and barriers', Journal of Consulting and Clinical. Psychology, 58, 4, pp. 425-31.

Peterson, L et al. (1988) 'Community interventions in children's injury prevention: differing costs and differing benefits', Community Psychology, 16, pp. 188-204.

Phillips, C J and Prowle, M J (1993) 'Economics of a reduction in smoking: case study from Heartbeat Wales', Journal of Epidemiology and Community Hea.th, 47, pp. 215-223.

Plotnick, R D (1994) 'Applying benefit-cost analysis to substance use prevention programs', International Journal of the Addictions, 29, 3, pp. 339-359.

Powell, M (1990) Reducing the costs of alcohol in the workplace: the case for employer policies, Discussion Paper 68, Centre for Heal.th Economics, University of York.

Rovira, J (1990) 'Economics of prevention', in Drummond M.F and Davies, L (eds) AIDS: the challenge for economic analysis, Heal.th Service Management Centre, University of Birmingham.

Rutz, W et al. (1992) 'Cost-benefit analysis of an educational program for general practitioners by the Swedish Committee for the Prevention and Treatment of Depression', *Acta Psychiatrica Scandinavia,* 85, pp. 457-464.

Sarvela, P D and Ford, T D (1993) 'An evaluation of a substance abuse education program for Mississippi Delta pregnant adolescents', *Journal of School Health,* 63, 3, pp. 147-152.

Scott, A I F and Freeman, C P L (1992) 'Edinburgh primary care depression study: treatment outcome, patient satisfaction and cost after 16 weeks, *British Medical Journal.*. 304, 883-887.

Shephard, R J (1992) 'A critical analysis of work-site fitness programs and their postulated economic benefits', *Medicine and Science in Sports and Exercise,* 24, 3, pp. 354-370.

Soderlund, N et al. (1993) 'The costs of HIV prevention strategies in developing countries', *Bulletin of the World Health Organisation,* 71, 5, pp. 595-604.

Tillgren, P et al. (1993) 'Cost-effectiveness of a tobacco 'Quit and Win' contest in Sweden', *Health Policy,* 26, pp. 43-53.

Tolley, K and Rowland, N (1991) 'Identification of alcohol-related problems in a general hospital setting: a cost-effectiveness evaluation', *British Journal. of Addiction,* 86, pp. 429-438.

Wagner, E H et al. (1994) 'Preventing disability and falls in older adults: a population-based randomized trial', *American Journal of Public Health,* 84, 11, pp. 1800-1806.

Woodward, R (1993) 'Evaluating the Wirral Health Mind project: Looking at information uptake and participants' responses', in Trent, D.R and Reed, C *Promotion of mental health: Volume 2-1992,* Avebury, Aldershot.

Other References

Albee, G W (1990) 'Suffer the little children', *Journal of Primary Prevention*, 11, 1, pp. 69-82.

Allied Dunbar Fitness Survey (1992) *A report on activity patterns and fitness levels*, Sports Council and Health Education Authority, London.

Allon, N (1982) 'The stigma of overweight in everyday life', in Wolman, B.B (ed.) *Psychological aspects of obesity: a handbook*, Van Nostrand Reinhold Co., New York.

Altman, D G 'The cost-effectiveness of three smoking cessation programs', *American Journal of Public Health*, 77, pp. 162-165.

Anderson, J P et al. (1986) 'Policy space areas and properties of benefit-cost/utility analysis', *Journal of the American Medical Association*, 255, pp. 794-795.

Andulis, D P and Weslowski, V B (1992) 'Health services needs and related costs for HIV care', *PharmacoEconomics*, 1, 2, pp. 79-83.

Bagert-Drowns, R L (1988) 'The effects of school-based substance abuse education - a meta-analysis', *Journal of Drug Education*, 18, 3, pp. 243-264.

Barker, C et al. (1993) 'You in mind: A preventive mental health television series', *British Journal of Clinical Psychology*, 32, pp. 281-93.

Barry, P B and DeFriese, G H (1990) 'Cost-benefit and cost-effectiveness analysis for health promotion programs', *American Journal of Health Promotion*, 4, 6, pp. 448-452.

Bartecchi, C E et al. (1994) 'The human costs of tobacco use 1', *New England Journal of Medicine*, 330, pp. 907-912.

Becker, H K et al. (1992) 'Impact evaluation of drug abuse resistance education (DARE)', *Journal of Drug Education*, 22, 4, pp. 283-291.

Block, J E et al. (1987) 'Does exercise prevent osteoporosis?' *Journal of American Medical. Association*, 257, pp. 3115-3117.

Bloom, D E and Glied, S (1989) 'The evolution of AIDS economic research', *Health Policy*, 11, pp. 187-196.

Borowitz, M and Sheldon, T (1993) 'Controlling health care: from economic interventions to micro-clinical regulation', *Health Economics*, 2, pp. 201-204.

Bowling, A (1995) *Measuring disease: a review of disease specific quality of life measurement scales*, Open University Press, Buckingham.

Bowling, A (1991) *Measuring health: a review of quality of life measurement scales*, Open University Press, Milton Keynes.

Brooks, R G (1995) *Health status measurement: a perspective on change*, Macmillan, Basingstoke.

Bruvold, W H (1990) 'A meta-analysis of the California school-based risk education program', *Journal of Drug Education*, 20, 2, pp. 139-152.

115

Buck, D et al. (1996) *Performance indicators and health promotion targets,* Discussion Paper No. 150, Centre for Health Economics, University of York.

Canadian Task Force on the Periodic Health Examination (1990) 'Periodic health examination, 1990 update 2', *Canadian Medical Association Journal,* 142, pp. 1233-1238.

Canning, H and Mayer, J (1966) 'Obesity - its possible effect on college acceptance', *New England Journal of Medicine,* 275, pp. 352-354.

Caswell, S et al. (1990) 'Evaluation of a mass-media campaign for the primary prevention of alcohol-related problems', *Health Promotion International,* 5, 1, pp. 9-17.

Chapman, S (1992) 'Changes in adult cigarette consumption in 128 countries', *Tobacco Control,* 1, 4, pp. 281-284.

Charles, S and Webb, A (1986) *The economic approach to social policy,* Heinemann, London.

Coast, J (1996) 'Efficiency: the economic contribution to priority setting', in Coast, J et al. (eds) (1996) *Priority setting: the health care debate,* Wiley and Sons, London.

Coast, J and Donovan, J (1996) 'Conflict, complexity and confusion: the context for priority setting', in Coast, J et al. (eds) (1996) *Priority setting: the health care debate,* Wiley and Sons, London.

Coast, J et al. (eds) (1996) *Priority setting: the health care debate,* Wiley and Sons, London.

Coast, J et al. (1996) 'An equitable basis for priority setting', in Coast, J et al. (eds) (1996) *Priority setting: the health care debate,* Wiley and Sons, London.

Coggans, N et al. (1991) 'The impact of school-based drug education', *British Journal of Addiction,* 86, pp. 1099-1109.

Cohen, D (1995) 'Messages from Mid-Glamorgan: a multi-programme experiment with marginal analysis', *Health Policy,* 33, 2, pp.147-156.

Cohen, D (1994a) 'Marginal analysis in practice: an alternative to needs assessment for contracting health care', *British Medical Journal.* 309, pp. 781-784.

Cohen, D (1994b), 'Health promotion and cost-effectiveness', *Health Promotion International,* 9, 4, pp. 281-287.

Cohen, D (1992) 'Using economics in health promotion', in Bunton, R and Macdonald, G (eds) *Health promotion: disciplines and diversity,* Routledge, London.

Cohen, D (1984) *Economic consequences of a non-smoking generation,* Health Economics Research Unit Discussion Paper 06/84, University of Aberdeen.

Cohen, D and Fowler, G (1993) 'Economic implications of smoking cessation therapies: a review of economic appraisals', *PharmacoEconomics*, 4, 5, pp. 331-344.

Cohen, D and Henderson, J (1988) *Health, prevention and economics*, Oxford University Press, Oxford.

Colditz, G A (1990) 'The economic costs of obesity', *American Journal of Clinical Nutrition*, 55, pp. 503S-507S.

Coyle, D and Tolley, K (1992) 'The discounting of health benefits in the pharamco-economic analysis of drug therapies: an issue for debate?' *PharmacoEconomics*, 2, 2, pp. 153-162.

Craig, N et al. (1995) 'Clearing the fog on the Tyne: programme budgeting in Newcastle and North Tyneside Health Authority', *Health Policy*, 33, 2, pp. 107-126.

Cribb, A and Haycox, A (1989) 'Economic analysis of the evaluation of health promotion', *Community Medicine*, 11, pp. 299-305.

Cummings, S R et al. (1989) 'The cost effectiveness of counselling smokers to quit', *Journal of the American Medical Association*, 261, pp. 75-79.

Dasgupta, A K and Pearce, D W (1974) *Cost benefit analysis: theory and practice*, Macmillan, Basingstoke.

Doll, R et al. (1994) 'Mortality in relation to smoking: 40 years' observation on male British doctors', *British Medical Journal.* 309, pp. 901-910.

Donaldson, C (1995) 'Economics, public health and health care purchasing: reinventing the wheel?' *Health Policy*, 33, 2, pp. 77-90.

Donaldson, C et al. (1995) 'Willingness to pay for antenatal screening carrier screening for cystic fibrosis', *Health Economics*, 4, pp. 439-452.

Donaldson, C and Gerard, K (1993) *Economics of health care financing: the visible hand*, Macmillan, Basingstoke.

Donaldson, S I et al. (1994) 'Testing the generalizability of intervening mechanism theories: understanding the effects of adolescent drug use prevention interventions', *Journal of Behavioral Medicine*, 17, 2, pp. 195-216.

Drummond, M F (1992a) 'The role and importance of quality of life measurements in economic evaluations', *British Journal of Medical Economics*, 4, pp. 9-16.

Drummond, M F (1992b) 'Cost-of-illness studies: a major headache?' *PharmacoEconomics*, 2, 1, pp. 1-4.

Drummond, M F (1989) 'Output measurement for resource allocation decisions in health care', *Oxford Review of Economic Policy*, 5, 1, pp. 59-74.

Drummond, M F and Davies, L (1990) *AIDS: the challenge for economic analysis*, Health Service Management Centre, University of Birmingham.

117

Drummond, M F et al. (1993a) 'Standardizing methodologies for economic evaluation in health care', *International Journal of Technology Assessment in Health Care*, 9, 1, pp. 26-36.

Drummond, M F et al. (1993b) 'Cost-effectiveness league tables: more harm than good?' *Social Science and Medicine*, 37, 1, pp. 33-40.

Drummond, M F et al. (1987) *Methods for the economic evaluation of health care programmes*, Oxford University Press, Oxford.

Ebrahim, S and Williams, J (1992) 'Assessing the effects of a health promotion programme for elderly people', *Journal of Public Health Medicine*, 14, 2, pp. 199-205.

Eisenberg, L (1992) 'Treating depression and anxiety in primary care: closing the gap between knowledge and practice', *New England Journal of Medicine*, 326, pp. 1080-1084.

Elixhauser, A (1990) 'The costs of smoking and the cost effectiveness of smoking-cessation programs', *Journal of Public Health Policy*, Summer, pp. 218-237.

Ellickson, P L et al. (1993) 'Preventing adolescent drug use: long-term results of a junior high program', *American Journal of Public Health*, 83, 6, pp. 856-861.

Elwood, P C et al. (1993) 'Exercise, fibrogen and other risk factors for ischaemic heart disease', *British Heart Journal.* 69, pp. 183-187.

Engleman, S R and Forbes, J (1986) 'Economic aspects of health education', *Social Science and Medicine*, 22, pp. 443-458.

Ennett, S T et al. (1994) 'How effective is drug abuse education? A meta-analysis of Project DARE outcome evaluations', *American Journal of Public Health*, 84, 9, pp. 1394-1401.

Ensor, T and Godfrey, C (1993) 'Modelling the interactions between al.cohol, crime and the criminal justice system', *Addiction*, 88, pp. 477-487.

Enzi, G (1994) 'Socioeconomic consequences of obesity: the effect of obesity on the individual', *PharmacoEconomics*, 5, (suppl.1), pp. 54-57.

Erickson, P et al. (1995) 'Operational aspects of quality-of-life assessment: choosing the right instrument', *PharmacoEconomics*, 7, 1, pp. 39-48.

Ershoff, D H et al. (1990) 'Pregnancy and medical cost outcomes of a self-help prenatal smoking cessation program in a HMO', *Public Health Reports*, 105, pp. 340-347.

Frankel, S and West, R R (eds) (1992) *Why wait? Tackling waiting lists in the NHS*, Macmillan, Basingstoke.

Freemantle, N et al. (1993) 'Managing depression in primary care', *Quality in Health Care*, 2, pp. 58-62.

Fries, J F et al. (1994) 'Randomized controlled trial. of cost reduction from a health education program: The California Public Employees' Retirement

System (PERS) Study', *American Journal of Health Promotion*, 8, 3, pp. 216-223.

Fries, J F et al. (1993) 'Reducing health care costs by reducing the need and demand for medical services', *New England Journal of Medicine*, 329, 5, pp. 321-325.

Fries, J F et al. (1989) 'Health promotion and the compression of morbidity', *Lancet*, 289, pp. 481-483.

Gerard, K (1992) 'Cost-utility in practice: a policy maker's guide to the state of the art', *Health Policy*, 21, pp. 249-279.

Godfrey, C (1993) 'Is prevention better than cure?' in Drummond, M F and Maynard, A (eds) *Purchasing and providing cost-effective health care*, Churchill Livingstone, Edinburgh.

Godfrey, C and Maynard, A (1992) *A health strategy for alcohol: setting targets and choosing policies*, YARTIC Occassional Paper 1, Centre for Health Economics, University of York, York.

Godfrey, C and Hardman, G (1990) *Updating the social costs of alcohol misuse*, Report to the Department of Health, Centre for Health Economics, University of York, York.

Godfrey, C et al. (1992) 'The economics of promoting sexual health', in Curtis, H (ed) *Promoting sexual. health,* [proceedings of the second international workshop on prevention of sexual transmission of HIV and other sexually transmitted diseases, Cambridge, March 1991], Health Education Authority, London.

Godfrey, C et al. (1989) *Priorities for health promotion: an economic approach*, Discussion Paper 59, Centre for Health Economics, University of York, York.

Goodin, R E (1982) 'Discounting discounting', *Journal of Public Policy*, 2, pp. 53-72.

Gorstein, J and Grosse, R N (1994) 'The indirect costs of obesity to society', *PharmacoEconomics*, 5, suppl.1, pp. 58-61.

Gortmaker, S L et al. (1993) 'Social and economic consequences of adolescence and young adulthood', *New England Journal of Medicine*, 329, pp. 1008-1012.

Grant, M (1989) 'Controlling alcohol abuse', in Robinson, D et al. (eds.) *Controlling legal. addictions*, Macmillan, Basingstoke.

Green, J J and Kelley, J M (1989) 'Evaluating the effectiveness of a school drug and alcohol prevention curriculum: a new look at "Here's looking at you, two"', *Journal of Drug Education*, 19, 2, pp. 117-132.

Hall, M (1994) *The impact of behavioural and biomedical advance on health trends over the next 25 years*, OHE Briefing No. 31, Office of Health Economics, London.

Health Education Authority (1991) *The smoking epidemic: counting the cost in Wales*, Health Education Authority, London.

Higgins, C W (1988) 'The economics of health promotion', *Health Val.ues*, 12, 5, pp. 39-45.

Hingson, R and Howland, J (1993) 'Alcohol and non-traffic unintended injuries', *Addiction*, 88, pp. 877-883.

Hjalmarson, A.I 'Effect of nicotine chewing gum in smoking cessation: a randomised placebo controlled double blind study', *Journal of the American Medical Society*, 252, pp. 2835-2838.

Hodgson, R et al. (1996) 'Effective mental health promotion: a literature review', *Health Education Journal.* 55, pp. 55-74.

Hodgson, T A (1994) 'Cost of illness in cost effectiveness analysis: a review of the methodology', *PharmacoEconomics*, 6, 6, pp. 536-552.

Hopkins, A (ed) (1992) *Measures of the quality of life and the uses to which such measures may be put*, Royal College of Physicians, London.

Hopkins, A (1990) *Measuring the quality of medical care*, Royal College of Physicians, London.

Hosman, C M H and Veltman, N (1994) *Prevention in mental health*, Dutch Centre for Health Promotion and Health Education, Utrecht.

Hu, T-W et al. (1995) 'The demand for cigarettes in California and behavioural risk factors', *Health Economics*, 4, 1, pp. 7-24.

Hughes, J et al. (1989) 'Nicotine versus placebo gum in general practice', *Journal of the American Medical Society*, 266, pp. 3133-3138.

Hunter, D (1993) *Rationing dilemmas in health care*, NAHAT Paper 8, Birmingham.

Jenkins, R (1993) 'Mental health promotion in the workplace', in Trent, D R and Reed, C *Promotion of Mental Health Vol.2 [1992]*, Avebury, Aldershot.

Johannesson, M et al. (1996) 'Outcome measurement in economic evaluation', *Health Economics,* 5, pp. 279-96.

Johannesson, M and Jonsson, B (1991) 'Economic evaluation in health care: is there a role for cost benefit analysis?' *Health Policy*, 17, pp. 1-23.

Jones, H G (1979) 'Allocation of resources' in Morris, D (ed) *The economic system in the UK*, Oxford University Press, Oxford.

Kaplan, R M (1988) 'New health promotion initiatives: the general. health policy model', *Health Promotion*, 3, 1, pp. 35-49.

Kaplan, R M and Davies, W K (1986) 'Evaluating the costs and benefits of out-patient diabetes education and nutrition counselling', *Diabetes Care*, 9, 1, pp. 81-86.

Katz, D A and Welch, H G (1993) 'Discounting in cost-effectiveness analysis of healthcare programmes', *PharmacoEconomics*, 3, 4, pp. 276-285.

Kent, A and Bowyer, C (1992) 'When weight gets out of control', *Doctor*, May, pp. 48-49.

Kobelt, G (1996) *Health economics: an introduction to economic evaluation*, OHE, London.

Lambert, J and Carrin, G (1990) 'Direct and indirect costs of AIDS in Belgium: a preliminary analysis', in Schwefel, D et al. (eds) *Economic aspects of AIDS and HIV infection*, Springer-Verlag, Berlin.

Lee, P R and Moss, A R (1987) 'AIDS prevention: is cost-benefit analysis appropriate?' *Health Policy*, 8, pp. 193-196.

Leu, R E and Schaub, T (1985) 'More on the impact of smoking on medical care expenditures', *Social Science and Medicine*, 21, pp. 825-827.

Leu, R E and Schaub, T (1983) 'Does smoking increase medical care expenditures', *Social Science and Medicine*, 17, pp. 1907-1914.

Levine, G N and Balady G J (1993) 'The benefits and risks of exercise training: the exercise prescription', *Advances in Internal Medicine*, 38, pp. 57-79.

Luce, B R (1996) 'The use of technology assessment and disease management by managed care pharmacy in the US', at *6th Annual Conference on System Science in Health Care*, Barcelona, September.

Luce, B R and Elixhauser, A (1990) *Standards for socio-economic evaluation of health care products and services*, Springer-Verlag, Berlin.

Lynch, W D and Vickery, D M (1993) 'The potential impact of health promotion on health care utilization: an introduction to demand management', *American Journal of Health Promotion*, 8, 2, pp. 87-92.

Lynn, L A et al. (1992) 'The pharmacoeconomics of HIV disease', *PharmacoEconomics*, 1, 3, pp. 161-174.

MacKenzie, T D et al. (1994) 'The human costs of tobacco use 2', *New England Journal of Medicine*, 330, pp. 975-980.

Main, J et al. (1993) 'Purchasing care for people with HIV infection and AIDS', *Qual.ity in Health Care*, 2, pp. 53-57.

Malek, M (ed) (1994) *Setting priorities in health care*, Wiley and Sons, London.

Mason, J et al. (1993) 'Some guidelines on the use of cost effectiveness league tables', *British Medical Journal*. 306, pp. 570-572.

Mawhinney, B (1993) Parliamentary written answer, *House of Commons Official Report (Hansard)*, March 3, col. 167.

Maynard, A (1994) 'Prioritising health care - dreams and reality', in Malek, M (ed) (1994) *Setting priorities in health care*, Wiley and Sons, London.

Maynard, A (1993) 'Cost management: The economist's viewpoint', *British Journal of Psychiatry*, 163, (suppl. 20), pp. 7-13.

Maynard, A (1991) 'Developing the health care market', *Economic Journal,* 101, pp. 1277-1286.

Maynard, A (1989) 'The costs of addiction and the costs of control', in Robinson, D et al. (eds.) *Controlling legal addictions*, Macmillan, Basingstoke.

McGuire, A (1988) *The economics of health care: an introductory text*, Routledge and Kegan Paul, London.

Mishan, E J (1983) *Cost benefit analysis*, Allen and Unwin, London.

Mooney, G (1994) *Key issues in health economics*, Harvester Wheatsheaf, London.

Mooney, G (1986) *Economics, medicine and health care*, Harvester Wheatsheaf, London.

Mooney, G and Lange, M (1993) 'Ante-natal screening: what constitutes a 'benefit'?' *Social Science and Medicine*, 37, 7, pp. 873-878.

Mooney, G et al. (1992) *Priority setting in purchasing: some practical guidelines*, NAHAT, Birmingham.

Morton, A et al. (1993) 'The patient profile approach to assessing the cost of AIDS and HIV infection', *Journal of Public Health Medicine*, 15, 2, pp. 235-242.

Moskowitz, J L (1989) 'The primary prevention of alcohol problems: a critical review of the literature', *Journal of Studies on Alcohol*, 50, 1, pp. 54-88.

Normand, C (1994) 'Making priority setting a priority', in Malek, M (ed) (1994) *Setting priorities in health care*, Wiley and Sons, London.

Nutbeam, D et al. (1991) *The Heartbeat Wal.es No-smoking Intervention: an empirical study of the economic viability of a health promotion programme*, Heartbeat Wal.es Technical Report 22, Health Promotion Authority for Wales, Cardiff.

Nutbeam, D et al. (1990) 'Evaluation in health education: a review of progress, possibilities and problems', *Journal of Epidemiology and Community Health*, 44, pp. 83-89.

O'Brien, B and Viramaster, J L 'Willingness to pay: a valid and reliable measure of health state preference?' *Medical Decision Making*, 14, pp. 289-297.

Oster, G et al. (1986) 'Cost-effectiveness of nicotine gum as an adjunct to physician's advice against cigarette smoking', *Journal of the American Medical Association*, 256, pp. 1315-1318.

Ovretveit, J (1995) *Purchasing for health*, Open University Press, Buckingham.

Palfrey, C F et al. (1992) *Policy evaluation in the public sector*, Avebury, Aldershot.

Parsonage, M and Neuberger, H (1992) 'Discounting and health benefits', *Health Economics*, 1, pp. 71-79.

Pearce, D W (1981) *Cost benefit analysis*, Macmillan, Basingstoke.

Pelletier, K R (1991) 'A review and analysis of the health and cost-effective outcome studies of comprehensive health promotion and disease prevention programs', *American Journal of Health Promotion*, 5, 4, pp. 311-315.

Petrou, S et al. (1993) 'Technical problems in the construction and use of cost per QALY league tables', *PharmacoEconomics*, 3, pp. 345-353.

Phelps, C E (1992) *Health economics,* Harper Collins, New York.

Phillips, C J et al. (1994) *Evaluating health and social care,* Macmillan, Basingstoke.

Phillips, C J and Prowle, M J (1992) 'Evaluating a health campaign: the Heartbeat Wales no-smoking initiative', *Contemporary Wales*, 5, pp. 187-212.

Phillips, D et al. (1993) 'The economics of smoking: an overview of the international and New Zealand literature', *PharmacoEconomics*, 3, pp. 462-470.

Piot, P (1992) 'Epidemiological perspective: an overview of HIV/STDs/reproductive health in Europe', in Curtis, H (ed) *Promoting sexual. health,* [proceedings of the second international workshop on prevention of sexual transmission of HIV and other sexually transmitted diseases, Cambridge, March 1991], Health Education Authority, London.

Posnett, J and Street, A (1996) 'Programme budgeting and marginal analysis: an approach to priority setting in need of refinement', *Journal of Health Services Research and Policy*, 1, 3, pp. 147-153.

Redman, S et al. (1990) 'The role of mass media in changing health-related behaviour: a critical. appraisal of two models', *Health Promotion International,* 5, 1, pp. 85-101.

Reid, D et al. (1992) 'Choosing the most effective health promotion options for reducing a nation's smoking prevalence', *Tobacco Control*, 1, pp. 185-197.

Richmond, R et al. (1995) 'Controlled evaluation of a general practice-based brief intervention for excessive drinking', *Addiction*, 90, pp. 119-132.

Rosen M and Lindholm, L (1992) 'The neglected effects of lifestyle interventions in cost-effectiveness analysis', *Health Promotion International.* 7, 3, pp. 163-169.

Ross, M W and Rosser, B R S (1989) 'Education and AIDS risks: a review', *Health Education Research: Theory and Practice*, 4, 3, pp. 273-284.

Rowland, N and Maynard, A (1993) 'Standardized alcohol education: a hit or miss affair?' *Health Promotion International.* 8, 1, pp. 5-12.

Royal College of Physicians (1995) *Setting priorities in health care,* Royal College of Physicians, London.

Royal College of Physicians (1977) *Smoking or Health,* Pitman Medical. London.

Rundall, T G and Bruvold, W H (1988) 'A meta-analysis of school based smoking and alcohol prevention programs', *Health Education Quarterly*, 15, 3, pp. 317-334.

Sackett, D et al. (1996) 'Evidence-based medicine: what it is and what it isn't' *British Medical Journal.* 312, pp. 71-72.

Schaapveld, K et al. (1990) *Setting priorities in prevention*, TNO Institute for Preventive Health Care, The Netherlands.

Segal, L and Richardson, J (1994) 'Economic framework for allocative efficiency in the health sector', *Australian Economic Review*, 2nd Quarter, pp. 89-98.

Schofield, P (1995) 'Accidents will happen but not quite so often', *Independent*, 23 February, pp.37.

Schwefel, D et al. (eds) (1990) *Economic aspects of AIDS and HIV infection*, Springer-Verlag, Berlin.

Scitovsky, A. (1989) 'The cost of AIDS: an agenda for research', *Health Policy*, 11, pp. 197-208.

Sheldon, T A et al. (1993) 'Examining the effectiveness of treatments for depression in general. practice', *Journal of Mental Health*, 2, pp. 141-156.

Shephard, R J (1987) 'The economics of prevention', *Health Policy*, 7, pp. 49-56.

Shipp, M et al. (1992) 'Estimation of the break-even point for smoking cessation programs in pregnancy', *American Journal of Public Health*, 92, pp. 383-390.

Smith, R (1992) 'Promoting sexual health: the best way to tackle HIV', *British Medical Journal.* 305, pp. 70-71.

Sonnenberg, P A and Beck, J R (1993) 'Markov models in medical decision making', *Medical Decision making,* 13, pp. 322-328.

St. Leger, A S (1989) 'Would a healthier population consume fewer health resources?' *International Journal of Epidemiology*, 18, pp. 306-311.

Sutherland, G et al. (1992) 'Randomised control trial of nasal nicotine spray in smoking cessation', *Lancet*, 340, pp. 324-329.

Sutton, M and Maynard, A (1994) *What is the size and nature of the 'drug' problem in the UK?* YARTIC Occassional Paper 3, Centre for Health Economics, University of York, York.

Thompson, M S (1986) 'Willingness to pay and accept risks to cure chronic disease', *American Journal of Public Health*, 76, pp. 392-396.

Thompson, R and Pudney, M (1990) *Mental illness - the fundamental facts*, Mental Health Foundation, London.

Ting, D and Carter, J H (1992) 'Behavioural change through empowerment: prevention of AIDS', *Journal of the National Medical Association, 84, 3, pp. 225-228.*

Tolley, K (1993) *Health promotion: how to measure cost-effectiveness*, Health Education Authority, London.

Tolley, K and Gyldmark, M (1993) 'The treatment and care costs of people with HIV infection or AIDS: development of a standardised cost framework for Europe', *Health Policy*, 24, pp. 55-70.

Tones, B K (1992) 'Measuring success in health promotion: selecting indicators of performance', *Hygie*, 11, pp. 10-14.

Tones, B K et al. (1991) *Health Education: effectiveness and efficiency*, Chapman Hall, London.

Townsend, J et al. (1994) 'Cigarette smoking by socioeconomic group, sex and age: effects of price, income and health publicity', *British Medical Journal*. 308, pp. 21-26.

Tsevat, J (1992) 'Impact and cost-effectiveness of smoking interventions', *American Journal of Medicine*, 93 (suppl. 1A), pp. 43-47.

Twaddle, S and Walker, A (1995) 'Programme budgeting and marginal analysis: application within programmes to assist purchasing in Greater Glasgow Health Board', *Health Policy*, 33, 2, pp. 91-106.

Vaandrager, H W et al. (1993) 'A four-step health promotion approach for changing dietary patterns in Europe', *European Journal of Public Health*, 3, pp. 193-198.

Wagstaff, A and Maynard, A (1988) *Economic aspects of the illicit drug market and drug enforcement policies in the United Kingdom*, Home Office Research Report No. 95, HMSO, London.

Warner, K E et al. (1988) 'Economic implications of workplace health promotion programs: review of the literature', *Journal of Occupational Medicine*, 30, 2, pp. 106-112.

Warner, M and Evans, W (1993) 'Pearls of wisdom', *Health Service Journal,* September 16.

Weinstein, M C (1990) 'Principles of cost-effectiveness resource allocation in health care organisations', *International Journal of Technology Assessment in Health Care*, 6, pp. 93-103.

Wells, N (1988) *HIV and AIDS in the United Kingdom*, OHE Briefing No. 23, Office of Health Economics, London.

West, R R (1996) 'Discounting the future: influence of the economic model', *Journal of Epidemiology and Community Health,* 50, pp. 239-244.

West, R (1994a) *Eating disorders: anorexia nervosa and bulimia nervosa*, Office of Health Economics, London.

West, R (1994b) *Obesity*, Office of Health Economics, London.

West, R (1992) *Depression*, Office of Health Economics, London.

Whelan, A et al. (1993) *Performance indicators in health promotion: a review of possibilities and problems*, Health Promotion Wales Technical Report No.2, Health Promotion Wales, Cardiff.

Wilde, G J (1993) 'Effects of mass media communication on health and safety habits: an overview of issues and evidence', *Addiction*, 88, pp. 983-996.

Wilkin, D (1992) *Measures of need and outcome for primary health care*, Oxford University Press, Oxford.

Williams, A (1995) *The measurement and valuation of health: a chronicle*, Discussion Paper No. 136, Centre for Health Economics, University of York, York.

Williams, A (1990) 'Ethics, clinical freedom and the doctors' role' in Culyer, A J et al. (eds) *Competition in health care*, Macmillan, Basingstoke.

Williams, A (1987) 'Screening for risk of CHD; is it a wise use of resources?' in Oliver, M et al. (eds) *Screening for risk of coronary heart disease*, Wiley, London.

Williams, A (1985) 'Economics of coronary artery bypass grafting', *British Medical Journal.* 291, pp. 326-329.

Williams, A (1981) 'Welfare economics and health status measurement', in Van der Gaag, J and Perlman, M (eds) *Health, Economics and Health Economics*, North Holland, London.

Windsor, R A et al. (1993) 'Health education for pregnant smokers: its behavioural impact and cost benefit', *American Journal of Public Health*, 83, 2, pp. 201-206.

Winn, S and Skelton, R (1992) 'HIV in the UK: problems of prevalence, sociological response and health education', *Social Science and Medicine*, 34, 6, pp. 697-707.

Wolf, A M and Colditz, G A (1994) 'The cost of obesity: the US perspective', *PharmacoEconomics*, 5, (suppl.1), pp. 34-37.